T0208337

To the Sufferer of this fatal disease
and their Devoted Caregivers my
Empathy and Sympathy.

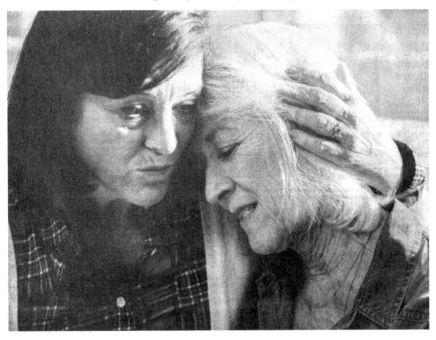

"For I am convinced that neither death nor life, neither angels nor demons, neither the present nor the future, nor any powers, neither height nor depth, nor anything else in all creation, will be able to separate us from the love of God that is in Christ Jesus our Lord".

(Romans 8:38-39, NIV)

Alzheimer's &Theology

Theological Dynamic of the Human Experience of Dementia

Thomas Liu, D. Min

Foreword by
Dr. Shiva Satish, M.D., Geriatricist

authorHOUSE®

AuthorHouse™
1663 Liberty Drive
Bloomington, IN 47403
www.authorhouse.com
Phone: 833-262-8899

Published by AuthorHouse 06/16/2021

ISBN: 978-1-6655-2732-3 (sc)
ISBN: 978-1-6655-2730-9 (hc)
ISBN: 978-1-6655-2731-6 (e)

Library of Congress Control Number: 2021910730

Print information available on the last page.

Holy Bible, New International Version®, NIV® Copyright ©1973, 1978, 1984,
2011 by Biblica, Inc.® Used by permission. All rights reserved worldwide.

Any people depicted in stock imagery provided by Getty Images are models,
and such images are being used for illustrative purposes only.
Certain stock imagery © Getty Images.

Photo Credit image on Title page: Houston Chronicle

This book is printed on acid-free paper.

ACKNOWLEDGEMENTS

This book, as with many things, was a collaborative effort of so many people who deserve thanks for their advice and their contribution to the intense process of writing. However, there are some for whom extra thanks is due. Particularly, I owe so much of what is written here to those people with dementia and their caregivers, with whom I had opportunities to communicate over many months in my capacity as a doctoral student and post-doctoral writer in pastoral-care theology. Reflecting back in many ways, I wonder how useful this book will be to readers in the future, as things might be different later than what I know now and what I will know later. As time passes, I hope it will be useful. For those who may already have passed on and have gone to be with the Lord, my precious memories of and experiences with you will live on. Special thanks to Dr. Jerry Terrill for his continuing encouragement, sharp comments, for taking time to read through and comment on earlier drafts and offering invaluable guidance, comment, and critique. I value very much both your thoughts and friendship. I am grateful also to Dr. Douglas Kennard with wonderful theological mind, for discussion regarding some of the underlining theological issues that permeate the book. I am grateful to staff from various memorial facilities (assisted living) for our conversations about the lives of people with severe intellectual disabilities. The stories of such people are not the same as those stories that are lived out by people with dementia, but the resonance is clearly there.

A tragic similarity exists between these two questions: "What does it mean to know God when one doesn't have the intellectual capacity to understand who God is?" and, "What does it mean to know God when one has forgotten who the Creator is?"

My sincere thanks to Dr. Silva Satish, MD for his long and deep experience as a geriatrist and his profound insights have helped me at various levels as I have wrestled with the complicated issues that emerge when reflecting theologically on the experience of dementia, also known as Alzheimer's Disease. I am grateful as well to Mr. Alex Carr of Washington University in Saint Louis, Missouri, at the Center for Alzheimer's Research, for investigating the *tau protein*, and for giving me important opportunities to share some of the research *material at the center. These experiences are invaluable in terms of shaping and forming this book.* To Dr. Kevin Hrebik, interim D. Min Specialization director at HGST to assist editing of the Script even he is busy ministering as chaplain in prison ministry. Most of all, I am eternally grateful to my family, especially my wife, Sue, the love of my life, for your endless patience and exhaustless support, my daughter, Debbie, son-in-law, Jack, and two grandsons, Jake and Jett, all of whom are inspirations and constant sources of confidence when life is filled with self-doubts. Finally, I am most appreciative of the Lord Jesus, for having perfect patience with me and remembering me when I have mindlessly forgotten who he is.

Yes, last but not least, I would like to acknowledge and offer my appreciation and gratitude to those authors, scholars and experts listed in the end notes for their contribution to this book pages after pages of their invaluable knowledge, information and expertise to the subject matter to complete the book.

CONTENTS

FOREWORD

When I was asked by my patient and friend, Dr. Thomas Liu, to review and write a Foreword for his book, initially I felt a little hesitant to accept his request. The word "theology" in the book title made me wonder if I was qualified to write anything pertaining to religion, especially about Christianity (I am not a Christian). Even if I were a Christian (Liu is a Presbyterian), but without having any formal training or education in a religious institute, I know I have limited Christian theological knowledge, and I feel inadequate to write a profound word to appreciate his work. But then as I was reading through his manuscript and it led me to understand what drove him to write this book. In his Introduction, he says that he is aging, which is true (he is 82 plus), and he knows that globally, especially many Americans in the States, are getting older and are poised on the brink of a "longevity revolution" because Americans are living longer and are healthier. As Baby Boomers come to age, more than one in five Americans will be over the age of 65. This will have a widespread impact on every aspect of society, which is already beginning to be felt. This impact has drawn Liu to work on this book and gave him the desire to help to relieve the sufferings of those who have been diagnosed with this dreaded brain disease and their caregivers who suffer along with the sufferers in their life journey. Basically, Liu says that it is God's love through Christ who encourages him to provide reason to hope in God's remembrance, hope that is from an informed theological perspective, a sense of purpose in the face of this disease and assurance that their condition is not leading to the end of their lives. Because of his godly motive and desire to offer help for those sufferers, it made it hard for me to refuse to accept his request.

As I have read through in the section, "Humanness and Personhood," Liu looks at different definitions of what constitutes a person with the question, "Who Am I?" He approaches dementia as a thoroughly theological condition. His basic premise is to fully understand the nature and experience of dementia, stating that the standard neurobiological explanations of dementia are deeply inadequate. He questions the notion that when people lose their memories they are no longer seen as the person they were before. Human beings are much more than bundles of memories; instead, their identity is tightly held in the memories of God.

The description of personhood in terms of purely human relationships also is not adequate. He writes, "The problem is that if it is our relationships that make up our personhood, then presumably if we don't have such relationships, we are no longer a person. But what about our relationship with God? To be a person is to be in You and I relationship, specifically with God. The security of human personhood is wholly determined by God.

This book provides abundance of practical information and informative, thoughtful, theological perspectives that provide a sense of purpose in the face of this disease. This is especially done by showing God's love to his crown creation—human beings—which were created according to his image and redeemed through the death and resurrection of Christ. He will protect them and will not forsake them whatever they may encounter, such as Alzheimer's Disease.

In this book, there are several stories of Alzheimer's from the patient's own point of view. Thoughts like biological determination are softened and made human so readers can encounter this personal narrative. Therefore, from my point of view, the book is targeted very much to mature audiences with some theological understanding. It would also be helpful for church pastors and caregivers of all kinds, but it could cross over into the academic world as curriculum for seminaries and ministers in training. I did have some problems grasping some of the theological content, but then that is a world in which I have yet to be immersed. For me, the strongest points of the book are the human and spiritual elements of Alzheimer's, per the subtitle, and I think those points will be what will attract those who are interested in this subject matter and can relate from these perspectives. These are what carry all the technical aspects, no different than the human side of hospital patients versus the medical aspects.

Therefore, I will put this book in the hands of my geriatric patients whom I think can benefit from reading it. I also think that it will be read gratefully by professionals, religious educators, and pastoral care church leadership. I will be turning its pages over and over again myself. Its marvelous readability makes "God cares" extremely accessible. Its integrity and depth makes every return to it very much worthwhile. This is a challenging, informative, thought provoking, and very readable text—such a help in changing thinking and attitudes towards dementia.

Shiva Satish, MD, Geriatrist

PREFACE

If the annual statistics concerning Alzheimer's Disease and dementia (hereafter it will be used interchangeably) are correct, more than six million people in the U.S. (50 million worldwide) suffer from various types of dementia, specifically to Alzheimer's disease, and those numbers are growing at an alarming rate. Based on current projections, by 2050, that number will exceed 16 million people (131.5 million worldwide), or about one in five Americans age 65 and older (I could easily be one of the them).

Alzheimer's takes a devastating emotional, financial, and physical toll on the families of those who are diagnosed with it. In 2016, nearly 16 million family members and friends provided more than 18 billion hours of unpaid caregiving assistance to those with Alzheimer's and other types of dementia. The cost of treating dementia worldwide hit an estimated $818 billion in 2015 and is rising by nearly 16% annually.

Aware of the broad impact of these illnesses, researchers have worked hard to find effective treatments. But dementia is an extremely complicated disease, with hundreds of clinical trials having failed, and some advances once thought to be promising have turned into dead ends. Several drug companies have stopped conducting research. A new approach is needed for funding solutions that improve the lives of older Americans. Only 12 years from now, the first millennials will be turning 49. Gen-Xers will begin turning 65, and the first Boomers will be turning 84, an age at which dementia is most prevalent. By that time, we can hope and pray that treatment and ultimately a cure for dementia can be added to the list of battles that have been won.

Meanwhile, from now to the time when the cure is discovered,

God continues to intervene. He says, "You are my people, created after my image and redeemed through the blood of my beloved Son Jesus. Whatever you may become I will protect you and I will not forsake you." Margaret Goodall once said,

> Anyone wishing to develop an understanding of dementia [needs to see it] from a Christian perspective, which offers hope based on experience and insight and encouragement to recognizing the darkness of dementia . . . [is] only a part of the story in which the person continues to be held in relationship by God who does not forget.[1]

Thus, if one day I, the author, would become a caregiver for one of my elderly family members who has been diagnosed with Alzheimer's disease, I probably will have no idea what the implications of this disease will be for us. In the months following the diagnosis, I may have to learn the hard way what are many of the tasks of caregiving. Probably no one in my family would be able to provide me with a coherent look at the full landscape of the caregiving task ahead, let alone the state of science and practical information I would need to meet these challenges. All the caregivers need hope . . . especially hope from an informed theological perspective that provides a sense of spiritual purpose in the face of this diseases; hope from medical science that sees return of function, not just adaptation as a feasible treatment goal; rather, hope in the form of someone simply willing to listen, to get into the deep water with both patients and caregivers. All types of hope, like real "cups of cold water" are needed to bond sufferers to professionals of all disciplines.[2]

Contrary to often misguided opinions, most families do not abandon the family members with disabilities (bodily or mentally) or terminal diseases and conditions to paid professionals and paraprofessionals. Yet most healthcare service practitioners and possibly some church leaders fail to acknowledge and affirm the central role that families play in extending caregiver services. This is because most people outside of professionals, including pastors and lay leaders, simply lack the necessary skills to encourage and enable families to do their Herculean jobs more effectively. Pastors and lay leaders especially need to acknowledge and support family caregivers in their vital role as a first step toward dealing with the growing phenomenon and unique challenges of family members caring for individuals with disabling conditions.

Many people who live in community settings, or who may belong to churches, require assistance at times because of chronic disease and disability, and dementia clearly is such a case of a common, chronic, and progressively disabling condition that affects both the person and the family. Following are definitions and details of what dementia is all about.

The term dementia (or senility) indicates a progressive, marked decline in intellectual or cognitive functions associated with damage to brain tissue. This may affect personality and behavior, and it may be either a reversible or an irreversible type. In the aging process, once there is loss of memory, the popular judgment is this must be the onset of the dreaded brain disease. Alzheimer's, which leaves the body still alive after the brain is dying or dead, is called neuropathic ideology. The current scientific culture holds intellect higher than love and emotional support, but there are two wonderful alternatives to drugs, one of which is diet and the other is love given in personal, loving, tender care.[3]

Lisa Genova, a neuroscientist with a Ph.D. from Harvard, wrote a moving novel (since made into a movie) titled *Still Alice* from a chillingly deterministic paradigm of genetics.[4] The subject, *Alice*, has a genetic deficiency that induces Alzheimer's disease, which then means one or more of her three children are also doomed to the same fate.[5] The book's setting is her alma mater, Harvard University. Alice has brilliant mind, but in mid-life her world suddenly crashed when she was diagnosed with an early onset form of Alzheimer's disease. Genova skillfully narrates Alice's progressive deterioration and her tortuous relationship with her daughter, Lydia. Make a long story short, even though Alice's neurological condition never improved, her relationship with her daughter eventually was restored.

The story of Alzheimer's from the patient's point of view, including biological determination and all aspects, is softened and made human when readers encounter this personal narrative. *Still Alice* leaves readers wondering about the values of our culture, questioning which is the worse atrophy—the loss of love in pursuit of academic ambitions or the loss of brain abilities from disease. There is tension between an unrelenting disease (embodied patient) and human (socialized person) care, encapsulated well by this statement by Oliver Sacks, a Columbia University Professor of neurology and psychiatry in New York, "In examining disease, we gain knowledge about anatomy and physiology and biology. In examining the person with disease, we gain wisdom about life."[6]

Whereas Alzheimer's may be specified as a brain disease, dementia is an encompassing concept that can be used theologically to reflect upon the deterioration of a much greater realm of personal stimuli, including one's social environment. A demented person may be said to have two forms of deterioration going on at the same time—a deterioration of the capacities of the brain to direct bodily functions and a diminishing social environment. These, indeed, comprise a multiplicity of personal losses. For Christians, dementia may also involve a loss of faith, a distancing or seeming absence of God, an empty prayer life, and other spiritually disquieting experiences.

Pioneering work on dementia care has been conducted by Tom Kitwood in such works as, "The New Culture of Dementia Care and Dementia Reconsidered: The Person Comes First,"[7] as well as other journal articles. Today, far better diagnostic skills and tools are in place for dementia, the scope of which has tripled in size and content. Laboring for a person is not equivalent to a cure, but an accurate diagnosis constitutes a necessary step in the right direction. Even so, major cultural modifications are still needed. Many seniors are confused about the terms dementia and Alzheimer's disease, and they still associate them with "no help," "no cure," and "no hope." Thus, a senior will now enter into a pattern of life that could include emotional and mental disarray, where it is often difficult to distinguish between cause and effect. Seniors rarely have the reflective power or the knowledgeable advice from others to face up to such issues. Categories of identity such as "senior," "patient," and "mentally ill," are all demeaning, yet they are consistent with a biological model of the human being.

In today's scientific culture, is there any greater threat to a senior than being told through various innuendos, "You are losing your mind"? The primary importance of loss of memory is a new universal fear among society's aging population for four primary reasons: 1) loss of their cognitive abilities, 2) significant personal changes, 3) concerns while interacting in society, and 4) the growing complexities of contemporary living. Into this setting, a Christian response speaks profoundly. Memory is far more intrinsically God's business than a human concern. As Julian of Norwich took up a small hazel nut into her hand, she said, "God made it, God cares for it; for God loves it!" It is God's character—the God who created human beings will take care of them even beyond the shadow of death. If a person knows that they came from a loving, healthy family, they can live confidently into the future. Biblically, we are assured that we were created, "in the image and likeness of God," and that his purpose was to be Immanuel, "God with us." Israel was assured God had made a covenant with them, to be "their God," who stipulated his bond with them as "the God who remembers" them. We can only fundamentally understand the category of personhood as a theological category, of being intrinsically relational in our creation by the infinite wisdom of the triune God of grace.

God had much more than a good memory. "God's remembrance" is a term that reflects his divine character in both redemption and judgment, his redemptive history of Israel. God's remembrance expresses his personal attentiveness towards his people, whether in grace or in judgment. Unlike human memory, which is corrupted and easily diverted to other loyalties, God's active remembering is identical with his actions and his character of love; it is at the heart of his creative and redemptive power. Our power of memory may not be sustained, but he is "the same yesterday, today, and forever" (Heb. 13:8).

Many passages in Scripture urge us to remember the Lord our God and his statutes. From the Hebrew context, Brevard Child states, "an act of remembrance in not a simple inner reflection, but involves an action, an encounter with historical events."[8] The past will not disappear so that we operate only presently, nor will God go away during our times of rebellion. Following the call to his exclusive attention, we should give ourselves completely to God, since our uniqueness reflects upon the universal human need of God, the relationship with him that no one else can rival. Such remembrance then is the equivalence of "choosing life," eternal life, over all else.

Biblical memory is always associated with heart, which is the most important anthropological metaphor in Old Testament. The heart functions to control all physical, mental, emotional, and spiritual functions. It is "the inner forum of the soul," the center of one's personal being in both its inner and outer realities."[9] Therefore, such "remembrance within the heart" is far deeper and richer than merely having a good memory. Significantly, a Christian in a state of advanced dementia, having lost mental memory, can remain secure in the Father's everlasting arms. God's unforgettable memory of us epitomizes his love for all humans, even if we are in an advanced state of dementia.

Unlike classical memory, which is merely the recall of reflective reason, at its best, Christian memory is recalling the existence of God and the belief that the soul itself is divine. Conjoining memory with the heart, the great Christian father of the church, Augustine of Hippo, sees memory as "the eye of the heart," and "the love of God" as the purpose of memory. In his beginning of *Confession*, "remembering the Creator" is the act of conversion and in praise of the heart, as in knowing the proper relationship to God. This then leads to the proper relationship with one's neighbor, or "other," to love socially as well. While memory plays a cognitive part for Augustine, as it must do, this is subsidiary to the interiority of personal relatedness to and with God, which lies at the heart of biblical faith.

The Reformation father, John Calvin, interpreted the Scriptures not as timeless truths but as the participatory engagement of God with human persons. It is by having a heart submissive to God, in the light of Christ, by the operation of his Holy Spirit, that we properly exercise the role of memory. So, memory is not the simple deposit of information we can recall later, but it is more truly the inward formation of the person being brought into relationship with the Trinity. Thus, there is no true memory for Calvin without God being its object in spiritual attentiveness.

So the autonomous self, which today is so threatened by the calamity of dementia, is itself "demented," for it has no true knowledge of one's self, nor indeed any knowledge of God.[10]

In his commentary on Deuteronomy, Calvin reminds us of God's remedy of remembrance: "Nothing but the recollection of [the Israelite] deliverance could tame their arrogance: for what could be more unreasonable than that they should be insolent who were formerly the slaves of a most haughty nation [Egypt], and who had not acquired their liberty by their own efforts, but contrary to their hope and deserts had obtained it by God's mere favor."[11]

Christian families dealing with dementia and other forms of mental deficiency can be assure and comforted that Christian faith is neither undermined nor destroyed by the losses of cognition. Primarily, God is mindful of his creation—not the other way around—as the Psalmist exclaims with gratitude and wonder in Psalm 8. Since our memory of God is much more a "soulful affair" than a matter of brain chemistry, the finding of neuroscience will never threaten our faith.[12]

Two-time Pulitzer Prize winner and Harvard biologist, Edward Wilson, is calling for a renewed partnership between religion and science in the hope of saving the earth. Yet, in this era of collaboration, many believers are troubled by the proliferation of academic efforts that appear to secularize faith and force a false, conventional religious consensus. Others are concerned about pejorative characterizations of their religion, particularly when such associations result in a loss of religious identity, community, and purpose. This book represents an effort to rejoin science and religion in ways that most positively impact the partnership. Our worldview informs and shape our lives. It influences a person's values, ethics, and capacities, and it directs our life trajectories, despite the scientific claim of objectivity.

Although faith is of divine origin, I, the author still open to what science aims to accomplish, which is to describe truth truthfully. With current widespread realities like healthcare chaplaincy, science has been more open to the responsible measurement and practice of religion and spirituality in matters of health. My hope is that the partnership will rise up and together find a cure for those who have suffered with such a horrible disease as Alzheimer's—not only for the patients but their caregivers. I am also hopeful that, with God's merciful grace and his intervention, we can all look forward for the day when prevention, care, and eventual cure will become a reality.

INTRODUCTION

Being Loved and Cared for
Who I May Become

"Neither height nor depth, nor anything else in all creation, will be able to separate us from the love of God that is in Christ Jesus our Lord" (Romans 8:39).

"The bottom line is—I'm in God's hands . . . and the medical community's. And hopefully they are in God's hands." Butch Noonan, *A Person with Dementia*[13]

At eighty-two plus years old, I am not getting any younger. Similarly, Americans as a group are also getting older. In fact, America is poised on the brink of a "longevity revolution"; we are living longer and healthier thanks in part to public health advances and medical research breakthroughs. The graying of the huge Baby Boom generation during the coming decades will amplify this fact with 20% of Americans being over the age of 65. These facts have numerous impacts on every aspect of society that are only beginning to be felt—from education, politics, economic, health, and certainly to religious institutions and churches. What draws me at my age to write this book? The answer is that I have the desire to help mitigate the sufferings of those who have been diagnosed with this dreaded brain disease, along with their caregivers who suffer alongside the sufferers in their life's journey. Fundamentally, it is God's love through Christ that encourages me to provide reasons to hope in God's remembrance, hope from an informed theological perspective, hope that provides a sense of purpose in the face of this disease and assurance that their condition is not leading to the end of their lives. Following is the Mission Statement of Lutheran General Hospital:

> Human ecology is the understanding and care of human beings as whole persons in light of their relationship with God, themselves, their families and the society in which they live.

Because of my advanced age, many thoughtless incidents have evidenced much of my own "forgetfulness," and often I would suspect that I might have contracted that disease. Because of this thought, it brings me to ask myself this unwanted question, "If I end up having Alzheimer's, how would I like to be treated?" The complicated answer to the simple question, however, is also the most distracting to me as I undertake such a complicated and sometimes difficult discussion about the theological dynamics of the human experience of dementia. In other words, if the question can be stated in different way such as, "If I—the author—have contracted dementia, I hope that I will be loved and cared for just for *who I am*, even if who *I become* makes it difficult to reconcile *who I was*, both for me and for others."

So who is the person with dementia? What if this person has forgotten to who he is and even worse, what if this person no longer knows who God is?

Who Would I Actual Be?

This question gravely troubles me. The concern above—to be loved and cared for just for *"who I am"*—is composed with simple words, but their practical meaning is profoundly complicated. Then, my mind was drawn to John Swinton's book, *Dementia: Living in the Memory of God*[14] and one of Dietrich Bonheoffer's prison poems titled, "Who am I?" in which he voiced my own concern in this way:

Who am I? This or the Other?
Am I one person today and tomorrow another?
Am I both at once? A hypocrite before others,
And before myself a contemptibly woebegone weakling.
Who am I? They mock me, these lonely questions of mine.
Whoever I am, thou know, O God, I am yours.[15]

Bonheoffer's question strikes strangely true for many people today. In this modern age, people constantly try but often fail to discover who they are and persistently strive to re-invent themselves because they assume that autonomous self-construction is a real possibility. While this question carries the weight of much cultural desire, the question is deceiving over its apparent simplicity. How can a person be the same today than they were twenty, thirty, and forty years ago? Over so many years, trillions of body cells have been replaced countless times. This person might still resemble their "previous self," but this person just does not look the same. Our thinking is not the same, nor are our priorities, values, desires, physical capacities, or psychological outlooks the same as when we were younger. Yet, despite the fact that there is little physical or psychological continuity between the "old-self" and the "new-self," both in fact are the same person. Laying out one's life in such ways, it is understandable and even normal that we may not be completely sure of just who we are at any given time.

Thus, the basic, common questions, "Who was I?" and "Who am I Now?" are complicated in the best of times. They would become infinitely more complicated if we were to develop dementia. Who will I be when I have forgotten who I think I am? Who will I become when that last tentative connection between who I thought I was then, and who I think I am now has been severed? What will they look like? If dementia leads a person to become a radically new "self," how could anyone expect people to love this stranger? Why would they? How could they? Who would they be loving? Who will they be? Yet this person wants and needs others to keep on loving them. This person does not want to be forgotten or abandoned. This person is not sure what it will look like to remember them when *they* have forgotten who they are . . . and who their God is. The Psalmist puts it this way, "Can the darkness speak of your wonderful deeds? Can anyone in the land of forgetfulness talk about your righteousness?" (Ps. 88:12).[16]

Love is a Many Splendor Thing

Genuine caring sprouts from true love, which is also quite a mysterious and complex thing. Remaining loved is not always the safest place to be. Some might seek to love the "Me-with-Alzheimer's" by offering comfort, solace, and friendship in my time of struggle. But others might see my Alzheimer's as a fate worse than death, and assumes that death would be a blessed release for me.[17] In the name of love and compassion, the person with Alzheimer's might seem to be a good reason for justifying euthanasia.[18] The person's loved ones might abandon them, because they think that they are no longer there, that they are already dead. The person's silent pleas, "It's still *ME*, Lord,"[19] may fall on deaf ears, leading them to feel like they are standing in the shoes of the Psalmist, crying out, "My loved ones and friends stay away, fearing my disease. Even my own family stands at a distance" (Ps. 38:11). Sadly, four out of five families take this way out, and two out of four families never again speak to the person. Perhaps, even if they can no longer speak with words, they will agree with the Psalmist's fateful resignation, "You have taken away my companions and loved ones. Darkness is my closest friend" (Ps. 8:18). When those days come, who will be the person's voice? Who will be the person's protector? Who will be the person's God?

What does it mean to love God and be loved by God when this (demented) person has forgotten who their God is? Then they might want to be careful about precisely what it means when they say they would like to be loved for who they are. Is it fair to ask to love a person even when the "that person" whom they used to love seems distant and perhaps even absent? If both primary needs—to love and be loved— no longer resemble what they *themselves* signed up for, how could this (demented) person expect others to love them as they always have before? As stated, it is a lot to ask others to remain faithful to them in the midst of their plight, and to continue to love them in the present as they have loved them in the past. How about the strangers who seek to care for this (demented) person when their family no longer can? The caregivers have never known this person apart from what they know them as now, a victim of Alzheimer's. What kind of love could such strangers give to this person . . . and this person to them? On the other hand, what would it be like if this stranger were treated as a child of God, knowing God still loves them, even for who they have become?

Loved by God

Despite by this person's own confusion, their identity, who they are, is known and held only by God. Bonheoffer's answer to the question, "Who am I?" is, "I am yours, God!" Here, he resonates with the prophet Jeremiah's affirmation that human identity is divinely shaped and held:

> But blessed are those who trust in the Lord
> And have made the Lord their hope and confidence.
> They are like trees planted along riverbank,
> With roots that reach deep into the water.
> Such trees are not bothered by the heat
> Or worried by long months of drought.
> Their leaves stay green
> And they never stop producing fruit.
> The Human heart is the most deceitful of all things
> And desperately wicked.
> But I, the Lord, search all hearts
> And examine secrete motives.
> I give all people their due rewards
> According to what their actions deserve. (Jer. 17:7–10)

In the end, only God knows who they are; only God searches their hearts and recognizes who they really are. God creates humans, sustains them, and knows them. Bonheoffer may well be correct in saying,

"Whoever I am, you know, God, I am yours!" Nothing can destroy such divine recognition, and here Bonheoffer finds peace. Perhaps here also, those suffering with Alzheimer's and those who accompany them on their journeys similarly can find peace. But what would such peace look like? What does it mean to be known, to be loved, and to be held by God when this person has forgotten who God is, and no longer can recognize themselves or those whom they once loved?

The core of the Christian argument and the heart of this book is related to developing a theological perspective specifically for Alzheimer's and dementia patients and their caregivers.

Dementia Is a Theological Condition

By seeing Alzheimer's as a theological condition, this script is firmly rooted within the Christian faith and engages with a wide range of disciplines. Such a perspective takes established knowledge seriously, but seeks to enable the discovery of opinions, possibilities, and perspectives that are crucial for a truly Christian understanding of Alzheimer's and the development of authentically Christian modes of Alzheimer's care. Therefore, such approaches to spirituality may well have their place within the overall arena of how human beings care of those whose lives are marked by Alzheimer's. This approach makes people aware of hidden dimensions of the experience of Alzheimer's and opens up important spiritual spaces within health and social care services, which have a tendency toward the secular and the mundane.[20] In fact, the focus will be on specific forms of spirituality and a theological understanding of the world that emerges from a perspective that is deeply informed by, although not uncritical of, the Christian tradition. This perspective presumes that the world was created by God, broken by sin, and is in the process of being redeemed through the saving works of Jesus.

The basic premise provides this writing with a particular orientation and dynamic and presents the relationship between theology and the other disciplines involved in the diagnosis and care of Alzheimer's in a particular way. Here I, the author, do not focus on how medicine can use theology to bring benefits to patients with Alzheimer's, which dynamic is quite different, and wrong-headed. For instance, many of participants of the growing religion-and-health conversation in the U.S. and E.U. make a fundamental mistake in seeming to assume that the goals of religion should echo and contribute to the goals of medicine and culture.[21] If religion eases depression and anxiety, then it should be grafted in as a resource for modern medical approaches to care and intervention.[22] If it helps people cope better with suffering, then someone should seek to develop interventions that enable effective coping.[23] If forgiveness is good for someone's mental health, then it should be incorporated into therapy.[24] From this perspective, it might seem natural to assume that if theology can help enhance the well-being of people with Alzheimer's, someone should use it as an aspect of their current medical understanding and practice. What is rarely considered, however, is the fact that the goals of medicine and theology and their respective definitions of health and well-being may be significantly different. Grafting theology into the goals of medicine simply on the grounds of potential therapeutic benefit inevitably will lead to confusion, dissonance, distortion, and contradiction.

At a basic level, well-being within Christianity is not gauged by the presence or absence of illness or distress. Religious beliefs and practices may well have therapeutic benefits, but that is not their primary function or intention. Nor is the efficacy of a "spiritual intervention" theologically determined according to criteria such as reduced anxiety, better coping, or a reduction in depression, important as these things may be at a certain level. Theologically speaking, well-being has nothing to do with the absence or reduction of anything. It has to do with the presence of something: *the presence of God in a relationship*. Well-being, peace, health—what Scripture describes as *shalom*—has to do with presence of a specific God in particular places who engages in personal relationships with unique individuals for formative purposes.[25] Rather than alleviating anxiety and fear, the presence of such a God often brings on dissonance and psychological disequilibrium, but always for the purpose of the person's great well-being understood in redemptive and relational terms.[26]

This is not to suggest that there cannot and should not be a creative and healing conversation between medicine and theology. There is much that these two disciplines can learn from each other. It is the grounds upon which such a conversation should be built that is crucial. Some persons do not do *theological reflection on Alzheimer's within a medical, psychological, or neurological context*. In other words, these disciplines do not set the context into which theology speaks. Rather, theology provides an understanding of the basic context into which the medical sciences speak. *These disciplines are practiced within the context of creation and under the providential sovereignty of God.* This is so even if that theological context is not formally acknowledged.[27] If people truly are relational, dependent creatures, created by a God who remains steadfastly at the helm of creation, moving it toward its final destiny, then each person's neurological state in a strict sense is theological, and even scientific explorations of that neurobiology in a strict sense are pre-theological. Thus, in a real sense, *neurology is theology*.[28] It is in this sense that this book is to assume that dementia is a thoroughly theological condition. It makes a world of difference to suggest that dementia happens to people who are loved by God, who are made in God's image, and who reside within creation. The task of theology is to remind people of that distinction and to push their perception of Alzheimer's beyond what is expected from a strictly medical perspective and, instead, to steer them toward the surprising and the unexpected.

The Theology is Challenged

The primary proposition of this writing is that standard neurobiological explanations of Alzheimer's are deeply inadequate for a full understanding of the nature and experience of Alzheimer's. Not only does this script include the biological, psychological, and social dimensions of Alzheimer's, but it also understands and recognizes the critical theological aspects. Unless someone develops this "whole sight" then they can really understand what it means to be a person with Alzheimer's living in God's creation. David Keck, in his book, *Forgetting Whose We Are: Alzheimer's Disease and love of God*, describes Alzheimer's as the "theological disease."[29] He perceives Alzheimer's as differing from many other forms of disease insofar as, in his opinion, it erodes the very essence of self and raises profound existential questions about personhood, love, sin and salvation:

> This disease does differ from other example of disease, anguish, and death. The unusual situation of prolonged mental deterioration and the need for sustained caregiving over many years means that we can no longer presume the existence of the cognitive subject when we are thinking theologically.[30]

Keck asserts that the person, the cognitively aware "I," which is the central focus of much contemporary and historical theology, is not available or at least is radically revised within the lives of people in the advanced stages of Alzheimer's. Keck's observation is worth exploring. A good deal of theology (and indeed, much of worship activity) hinges on the assumption that theologians are addressing an individuated who is experiencing a cognitively able self, who is perceived as a reasoning, thinking, independent, decision-making entity. This cognitively able self is assumed to have the potential to know and understand certain things about God, a God who is available at an intellectual level through such things as revelation, prayer, observation, and other form of self-conscious spiritual experience.

Knowledge of God, sin, salvation, discipleship, sanctification, and justification, are all assumed to relate to a fully cognizant being who can understand certain things, who can avoid or engage in certain ways of thinking and acting, and who is able to make particular choices that have positive and negative implications and consequences for now and into eternity. Even at a basic level, the assertion, "If you confess with your mouth, 'Jesus is Lord,' and believe in your heart that God raised him from dead, you will be saved" (Rom. 10:10), requires a certain level of subjectivity, awareness, and cognitive competence. In this context, those whose intellect, condition, and memory have been devastated by dementia have a serious problem—how can they claim to love God when they have forgotten who God is?

Knowing God and Self

Focus on knowing God and emphasis on the cognitive self are common themes within theology. John Calvin, in his *Institutes of the Christian Religion*, states,

> Nearly all the wisdom which possess true and sound wisdom consists of two parts: the knowledge of God and of ourselves. But, while joined by many bonds, which one precedes and brings forth the other is not easy to discern.[31]

For Calvin, knowledge of God and knowledge of oneself (self-knowledge) are wholly intertwined. People can know who they are and why they have what they do only if they look at themselves in the light of God:

> no one can look upon himself without immediately turning his thought to the contemplation of God, in whom he "lives and moves" (Acts 17:28). For, quite clearly, the mighty gifts with which we are endowed are hardly from ourselves; indeed, our every being is nothing but subsistence in the one God. Then, by these benefits shed like dew from heaven upon us, we are led as by rivulets to the spring itself.[32]

As people recognize their dependency, their contingency, and their location within God, so they are freed to see their true state. As people come to know God, they discover who they are. The more they know of God, the more they realize the depth of their own depravity; the more they are drawn toward the wonder of God's grace and sanctifying love. Knowledge of God leads to worship and an awareness of who they are before God. The author has no quarrel with Calvin's suggestion regarding the contingent nature of human beings, since knowing God leads to worship. But it is easy to see problems when people apply Calvin's ideas about knowledge of God to the lives of those with Alzheimer's. If knowledge of God is necessary for knowledge of self, and if the only way to access someone's identity is through active contemplation of who God is, then they have problem. What happens when people can no longer remember either self or God. If people can no longer contemplate God? Will they then no longer know God? Augustine has a similar emphasis on the knowing of self:

> Great are you, O Lord, and exceedingly worthy of praise; Your power is immense, and your wisdom beyond reckoning. And so we men, who are a due part of your creation, long to praise you—we also carry our mortality about with us. . . . Anyone who invoked what is still unknown may make a mistake. Or should you be invoked first, so that we may then come to know you? But how can people call upon someone in whom they do not yet believe? But how can they believe without preacher, but Scripture tells us that those who seek the Lord will praise him. . . . My faith calls upon you, Lord, this faith which is your gift to me, which you have breathed into me through the humanity of your Son and the ministry of your preacher.[33]

If people's hearts are restless until they discover God, if the human vocation is to know and to worship God and nothing but God,[34] then at best, people with advanced Alzheimer's are destined to be eternally restless, and at worst, they are never going to find or rediscover the place of heart-to-heart peace within the heart of God. If finding God requires that people actively seek after him, then will those who no longer can remember what it might mean to do so find themselves trapped without the ability to praise God? If people cannot know and praise God, then how can their hearts be anything other than restless?

As Anselm suggests, faith has to do with seeking understanding—that is, "an active love of God seeking a deeper knowledge of God"—then it is clear that people with advanced Alzheimer's have no real way of finding God. The experience of seeking understanding is precisely of being lost as one encounters the latter stages of the process of Alzheimer's. It would appear that people who are losing their sense of self will struggle to access God, who appears to directly address only the cognitively able, and who offers no real way to access people for whom selfhood might have a radically different meaning.

Thus, even in theological ideas that at first might seem to lend themselves positively to the losses that accompany dementia, problems are present. Friedrich Schleiermacher argues that God is given and present in and with the feeling of "absolute dependence." As an existential experience that resonates in interesting ways with the experience of advanced Alzheimer's, discovering God in absolute dependence has the potential to be helpful. Absolute dependence is the true state of all human beings, and that radical dependence has important implications for how persons frame dementia. For Schleiermacher, the awareness of God is the *feeling* of absolute dependence:

> The feeling of absolute dependence, accordingly, is not
> to be explained as an awareness of the world's existence,
> but only as an awareness of the existence of God, as the
> absolute undivided unity.[35]

Such a feeling requires an awareness of the nature of God, and such awareness requires a person to have the cognitive capacity to develop the conceptual language necessary to be aware and to feel dependent on God. How does one know God when one cannot understand or conceptualize the meaning of absolute dependence or interpret and make sense of such a feeling? Despite the fact that the lives of people with advanced Alzheimer's are profoundly marked by the experience of "absolute dependence," this is not what Schleiermacher has in mind.

A Practical Theological Approach to Dementia

These theological problems are not simply dissociated "academic" arguments. They are in fact deeply practical in consequence and orientation. Keck notes,

> The loss of memory entails a loss of self, and we can no longer be secure in our notion of "self-fulfillment." Indeed, our entire sense of personhood and human purpose is challenged. Because we are dealing with the apparent disintegration of human beings—a thorough reconsideration of many fundamental theological questions is not entirely out of order.[36]

If the primary focus of theology is on the cognitively aware objective self, and if that very self is perceived to be dissolving as the process of Alzheimer's works itself out, then the forgetfulness that marks Alzheimer's inevitably will be mirrored by the ways in which theology forgets the experiences of people with Alzheimer's. This dual forgetfulness—one the product of neurology, the other the outcome of hyper-cognitive theological assumptions—inevitably will lead to practices that are ill-informed, theologically naïve, and potentially destructive. Keck is right in suggesting that what is required is a thorough reconsideration of some fundamental theological questions.

Keck's statement that the self is dissolved in the context of advancing Alzheimer's is in fact true. He is right, if people are their memories, if people sense of who and what they are in the world is determined by what they can remember about themselves and world around them—therefore, losing their memory will inevitably mean losing themselves. If we are to be perceived as so many isolated islands of memories, then we inevitably will disappear when these memories abandon us. In this sense, Alzheimer's does indeed seem to dissolve such people since it challenges every cultural assumption of a life well-lived. Human beings, however, are much more than bundles of memories. There is a world of difference between an *apparent* (Keck) dissolution of a human being and the *actual* dissolution of that person. There are many things seem *apparent* regarding people with Alzheimer's, but if one goes deeper, if one listens to people and is prepared to give them the benefit of the doubt, that which at first seems *apparent* is quickly revealed to be much more complex, opaque, and surprising. It is true when we encounter people with Alzheimer's, we no longer can be secure in our notions of self and self-fulfillment, but that is at least partly because such notions may be false perceptions based on false premises. It will be one of the tasks here to show that, devastating as Alzheimer's undoubtedly is, the human beings who experience it do not dissolve. They are certainly changed, and there is much suffering and cause for lament, *but these people remain tightly held within the memories of God.* In reality, the pure ideas about what humanness, the nature of the self, and self-fulfillment mean are what must be dissolved and re-created.

In giving voice to certain key questions that arise in the context of the experience of Alzheimer's, particularly advanced Alzheimer's, the intention here is to provide a practical and theological re-orientation that moves beyond current tendencies to perceive the subjective, self-aware, cognitive self as the necessary qualification for humanness and theological construction, and to open up the possibility that knowing *about* God may not be as important as *knowing* God, and that knowing God involves much more than memory, intellect, and cognition.

1

Dementia: A Practical Theology on a Biblical Foundation

We are to attempt an answer to the question, "What is there within the Bible? What sort of house is it to which the Bible is the door? What sort of country is spread before our eyes when we throw the Bible open?"

—Karl Barth[37]

As a theological discipline, *practical theology* seeks to explore the interface between the practices of the church and the practices of the world with a view to enabling faithful participation in God's redemptive practice in, to, and for the world.[38] Practical theology is that aspect of theology which seeks to bring together theology and practice in an attempt to describe the world, in order that the practices of Christians can remain true to the practices of God in, to, and for the world. Theology has to do with the knowledge *about* God, however, such knowledge is not simply intellectual. Knowledge about God should lead to, and indeed requires knowledge *of* God, which is necessarily experiential, practical, and transformative.[39] Theology provides a lens through which to look at the world. It offers a perspective on the way things are that scripts and guides Christian thinking, perception, and living. The object in this book is to use this lens to develop a theological redefining of dementia that is shaped by a different script. Such an approach acknowledges the pain and suffering that dementia brings to those diagnosed and their families, but it offers an alternative theological reading of the condition within which hope and new possibilities—in the present and for the future—remain even in the midst of deep forgetfulness. This different view of dementia will enable us to respond to it differently.

Redefinition as a Mode of Practical Theology

The central aspect of my approach can be described as "theological redescription." Walter Brueggemann, in his book *Redefining Reality: What We Do When We read the Bible*, proposes that the task of Scripture is not simply to offer moral guidance and tell us things about God, although it certainly does these things, but Scripture's task also is to *redefine the world*. The Christian's task is to enter into the strange world of the Bible and to allow that world to redefine reality for him or her. As people learn to live in this redefined world, they encounter God and one another in fresh and challenging ways and find the resources for faithful discipleship.[40]

Brueggemann argues that people make sense of the world by utilizing a variety of implicit and explicit scripts (stories that comprise our worldviews). These scripts help us to define, negotiate, act on, and make sense of the world. For example, nationalism, religion, capitalism, psychology, and biomedicine would be five primary scripts that form the epistemological context of Western liberal cultures. They are so powerfully and deeply ingrained in our thinking that we often do not recognize the impact that they have on the ways in which we see and understand the world, which includes the ways in which we see and understand Scripture. Most no longer recognize that these scripts have been taught to them by people and systems that have particular goals, intentions, and worldviews—which often are incongruous with Scripture and Christian theology.

However powerful and apparently decisive these defining scripts may seem to be, their claims are always open to *counterclaims* that may challenge or even overpower their definition of the way the world is. The

Christian narrative is one such counterclaim. Scripture calls the church to live by a different script, which emerges from within "the strange new world within the Bible.[41] This script offers a radical redefinition of the world, turning it from a place of individualism and competitiveness, a place where autonomy, freedom, and choice reign supreme, into a place where one discovers the sovereign and majesty of God who has created all things. In this new space of creation, people discover that salvation comes through brokenness,[42] strength comes through weakness,[43] and gentleness is revealed as an ontological aspect of the Messiah-who-is-God.[44] It is important to note that this strange world is a place where intellect and human wisdom are perceived as barriers rather than aids to faithfulness.[45] Inevitably, dementia will look different within such a new strange world. As such, the practical theological task will be one of offering a critical redefinition of the world in the light of the new script of the gospel. The task then is to *redefine the world* in the light of Scripture and tradition and to look carefully at what dementia looks like within this strange new world.

The World is Challenged

Brueggemann's point is similar to the point regarding the relationship between theology and medicine. To challenge the world, the Christian task is not to try to make the Bible relevant to society; it is quite the opposite. Christians are called to help society to recognize that it actually has already been living within the strange world that is defined in the Bible, but it has just forgotten this primal fact. The Bible is not just inspirational and hopeful; it is revelatory and transformative. Put in terms of intentions, its task is not simply to see how the Christian story can contribute to one's current understandings of dementia, although this certainly is important. The deeper task is to see what people's current understandings of dementia and practices that emerge from their worldview looks like when they are viewed and redefined from the perspective of the strange biblical world.

What does the Scriptures have to say about this disease? Let the emphatic Spirit answer and then explain for us what is said in the Bible, which is that the mind, the will, and the emotions are included in the soul. Brueggemann suggests that "every time the church takes up Scripture, it undertakes a serious challenge to dominant characterizations of our social world. It dares to propose an alternative reading of the world, an alternative version that is in fact a sub-version that rests beneath the dominant version in a less aggressive form."[46] Quoted from Psalms 119:105, "God's word is the *lamp* and *light* that guides people in the world." It redefines the basis of power and the nature of the world, about what the world is and how humans should function within it. The Bible reveals in fresh and radical ways the meaning of living well in sickness and in health.

To protect against negative and misleading definitions, seeking to redefine dementia using Scripture, theology, and tradition is insisting that "the initial presentation of reality is not an adequate or trustworthy account."[47] In contrast to the *cultural* definitive that underpins one's perception of being loved and desired, the basic assertion that people live in *biblical* creation offers a radical redefinition. Autonomy and freedom are meaningful only as they relate to the contingency of human beings before God. If God is the Creator, and if people live in a creation which God says is good,[48] then at the very least they know that they are created out of love and loved beyond all measure.[49] If God knew people when they were still in the womb (Ps. 139:13), and if God indeed has plans for them to prosper,[50] then neurological decline cannot separate them from the love of God and their ongoing vocation as human beings. *Lives that are touched by profound forms of dementia still have meaning and continuing purpose.*

The redefinition of dementia that is offered here will not, of course, be wholly independent of traditional definitions, which may turn out to be necessary but are insufficient. For example, regarding the resurrection of body (1 Cor. 15), the art of theological redefinition recognizes that the redefined world will have continuity and discontinuity with what has gone before. The old definitions retain some degree of utility and value but are transformed in important ways. The new definition, as Brueggemann explains, "employs in fresh ways speech that is already known and darling, venturesome ways that intensity, subvert, and amaze."[51]

The thoughts presented here critically serve to intensify and subvert the known and trusted scripts that have been constructed around the nature of dementia. Rather than simply uncritically reiterating the standard account of the disease, this work redefines the condition in ways that are recognizable but which become intense, subversive, and perhaps amazing as one encounters the radical scripts of Scripture, theology, and tradition. Such redefinition will enable dementia to look and indeed to be something quite different from its culturally constructed norms. This, in turn, will lead to responses that are caring, compassionate, and above all else, faithful.

In sum, the definition of redefinition will be provided as a practical theological method:

> Redefinition is an interdisciplinary approach to practical theology that seeks, in the light of Scripture and Christian tradition, to redefine objects, actions, situations, and contexts in ways that reveal hidden meanings, modes of oppression and misrepresentation, with a view to offering a fuller and more accurate description that highlights alternative understandings and previously inconceivable options for theory and actions.

The Stories that Are Told

Central to the approach of redefining concepts is the significance of the *stories that people tell*: "Who am I when I have forgotten who I am?" Relevant to that question is having the awareness that *people are the stories that they tell* about themselves and that are told about them. *Human beings are natural storytellers.* We live in a world that is profoundly shaped and formed by stories. From earliest known history, people have told stories about themselves and one another. People tell stories to identify themselves—stories about their past, their hoped-for futures, and what is happening in the here and now. People continually move backward and forward in time as they use their stories to describe who they were, who they are, and who they hope to become. Storytelling reveals the inherent timelessness of human existence. With just a few words, people can traverse years, racing backward toward their most important memories or shifting forward toward infinite possible futures. People perceive themselves as existing in the present, but at any given time a story can take them backward or forward in time, recalling or reframing old experiences or opening them to future worlds that contain possibilities they have not even considered before. Some of the stories people tell and that are told about them are true, some are embellished or imaginative, and others are just plain false. All of our stories, however, come together to give us a sense of who we are and where we are located at any given time within the ongoing meta-story of life.

The Impact of Counter-Stories

While a person's identity, in a sense, may change over time, they normally remain aware that certain stories—whether about themselves, others, or the world around them—are true and others are not. People can be mistaken or deceived, but they still continue to believe or disbelieve the stories. Even illusory stories, if people believe them, are true in their consequences. Under normal circumstances, most people are able to effectively negotiate their narrative worlds and gain and retain a more or less realistic sense of who they are. In whatever flawed way, they can articulate this sense of self-in-the-world in ways that present and maintain their identity within their public and personal realms. This in turn protects them from the imposition of false identities that may be inaccurate or dangerous. Because not all stories are true, some stories need to be countered. The key to holding onto one's identity, even if we are not entirely sure of who we are, lies in the art of being able to effectively tell counter-stories that correct the picture.[52] There, *the power of counter-stories* becomes highly relevant.

Tragic circumstances in life, such as dementia, often result in the loss of ability to tell one's own story. Once diagnosed with this disease, the ready availability of plausible, positive counter-stories is not always apparent. For people with dementia, the loss of storytelling ability is a gradual process. It is over a lifetime that stories both retain and shape our experiences and place the parameters on their identity, personhood, and experience. Those with advanced dementia, unfortunately, simply no longer have the ability to articulate counter-stories in ways that provide them with enough social power to sustain their identities as valuable and capable human beings.[53] The various stories told by the powerful others who surround them—doctors, neurologists, family, and friends—eventually overwhelm their own stories, which leaves them echoing author Christine Borden's words, "Who will I be when I die?"[54] and resonating in a strange way with Jesus' question to his disciples, "Who do you say I am?[55] Even if people with dementia have important stories to tell about themselves and others, who will listen? Gradually, the question changes from that which is asked by all people, "How can I tell my story well?" to a new and more complex question, "Who will tell my story well?' Having to ask the latter question puts people in a position of tremendous vulnerability. In a culture that prizes memory, intellect, freedom, reason, and autonomy, what kinds of stories will be told about those who seem to be losing such critical essences? Their question is haunting, "Who will tell their stories well when they have forgotten who they are?"

Revelation of Story and Counter-Story

A deeper question is how are the stories and counter-stories of dementia to be evaluated? Some of the central stories people have been accustomed to using to explain the phenomenon of dementia are at best inadequate and at worst deeply flawed. Like those with the disease, the disease itself also requires counter-stories that will correct, clarify, and update it in a trustworthy way. Even more significantly, people need to be able to redefine dementia in the light of the coming kingdom of God. One can argue that the Christian story offers strong possibilities in terms of the development of transformative counter-stories. When spoken into the experience of dementia, the Christian story has the potential to reveal and reframe dementia in vital ways. Such a counter-story offers a radical redefinition of the world and of dementia. It challenges accepted stories of biomedical determinism, inevitable neurological decline, the nature of suffering, the prioritization of the intellect, the role of memory, the potency of individualism, competitiveness, and autonomy, and the value of freedom. The counter-story of God does the work of repairing broken or misleading narratives and, as such, will become a place of rupture, resistance, and change. This new counter-story will not be read and understood apart from the old narrative. Neurology, psychology, biomedicine, and psychiatry remain vital aspects of dementia care, but they will be seen in a different light. Instead of providing a script that shapes and determines people's understanding of dementia, they themselves will be called to learn a new script.

Listening to Stories

Throughout, smaller, personal stories that also function to counter some of the more oppressive stories that surround dementia, one must bear in mind that while listening to them, the primary counter-story and substories of the gospel are indispensable. It would be a mistake to read these stories as simply illustrating the points that are being observed in patients, or as neutral foci for theological reflection. These stories are themselves strong counter-stories that will help to redefine dementia in important ways and will enable readers to see the practical relevance of the broader and wider counter-story of God's actions in the world. As someone engages with these stories, it will be helpful to keep in mind that each contains and reveals deep insights into the nature and character of God, and his practices in, to, and for humanity. As Karl Barth observes, "one cannot know God apart from that which God chooses to reveal," adding,

> *God is known only by God.* We do not know him, then, in virtue of the views and concepts with which in faith

we attempt to respond to his revelation. But we also do not know him without making use of his permission and obeying his command to undertake this attempt. The success of this understanding, and therefore the veracity of our human knowledge of God, consists in the fact that our viewing and conceiving are adopted and determined to participation the truth of God by God himself in grace.[56]

God is known only according to what he chooses to reveal. God is known as God acts. One way to frame these various stories is to say that there are places of revelation, places where God in some sense is acting and revealing. God acts in big stories in history—the Exodus, the Cross, and Redemption—but he also acts in and through the smaller stories of human life. Those who take time to listen and reflect can discover God's practices of revealing and acting in the strangest of places.

The Stranger in the Bible

Who are these strangers? Human beings once were strangers in God's eyes. In his essay, "The Stranger in the Bible," Elie Weisel draws attention to Jewish history and the significance of the stranger. He points out that the Hebrew Bible provides three terms for stranger: *ger, nochri,* and *zar.* The *gerim* (plural) were looked upon with favor and enjoyed unusual privileges; they adjusted and assimilated. They lived among the Jewish people, a community not originally their own or in a place not inherently his own; they adopted the Jewish faith, customs, and values, and made Jewish friends.[57]

The *gerim* were protected or dependent foreigners or strangers who had come among the people of God and had chosen to live with them. Thus, to love a stranger is to love a *ger,* someone who is worthy of respect, hospitality, and welcome. The people of Israel knew what it was like to be strangers, since they once were strangers themselves (Lev. 19:34, NKJV). As Jonathan Cohn points out, "We must treat others the way we have been treated. We must show them compassion, charity, and love. Above all, we must not make them feel like strangers."[58]

God raised up Israelites who belonged to the family of God and who were blessed when they remained true to God's promises. In the same way, the Jewish people were called to recognize their history as *gerim* and to treat *gerim* as God had treated them. It was not enough simply to include them within the community; *gerim* were to be made to feel welcome, to feel like they no longer were strangers.

Cohen and Wiesel open the biblical idea and help people's understanding of the strangeness of dementia by showing clearly that God is located in that place where the *ger* sojourns. The people of God at all times and in all places were to be people who accepted and welcomed the stranger. Continuing the biblical principle, Christians also are obligated to offer hospitality and welcome to the *ger*, because they belong to the same story and worship the same God. It brings fresh poignancy to Jesus's words in Matthew 25:35: "I was a stranger and you welcomed me."

Cohen applies this understanding to the lives of people with intellectual disabilities (dementia/Alzheimer's). He perceives them as modern-day *gerim* whom the church must not only incorporate but also receive as they would want to be received. Cohen argues that linking intellectually disabled people with the *gerim* helps one to understand the meaning of intellectual disability. God is with the *gerim*, and that reminds all people where God is and what it means to share a soul with God, and what it means to be a creature.[59]

Where Does Theology's Journey into Alzheimer's Begin?

To summarize, medicine (in the case of Alzheimer's, psychiatry), is a recognized tradition or set of traditions that produces its own forms of accepted knowledge and worldviews, which in turn leads to particular ways of looking at human beings and human experience. An impaired perspective on Alzheimer's is a natural outcome of the form that psychiatric medicine has adopted over time. There is nothing inherently wrong with this, and it is not to be perceived as anti-psychiatric. Such knowledge is important as a contribution to human wellbeing, and knowledge of the neurology of Alzheimer's is an important dimension of understanding it medically. To use the metaphor of Gilles Deleuze and Félix Guattari above, that aspect of the territory remains in place, although it requires significant modification. The emphasis on impairment, however, requires a degree of deterioration. The nature of medical knowledge and medical training means that those working within the field of mental health often are schooled to see some things and, by implication, not others. They are called to make sense of a cluster of human illnesses according to the particular theoretical frameworks by which they have been trained to see and describe their features. Thus, by definition, the specific focus of the professional gaze excludes certain things that may be vitally important. It is unlikely, for example, that such things as God, faithfulness, discipleship, sin, and love will emerge as part of any medical definition of any form of illness. Unhappiness and relational disconnection might, but sin and love? Such things are not being looked for, so they are not perceived as significant within the context. The fact that it might seem strange and counter intuitive to the reader to suggest that something like sin, love, the presence or absence of God might be a central part of a medical definition of Alzheimer's makes the point, and indicates the boundaries of medical diagnosis and the limited intentions that such a process has. Such an observation should alert people to be more than a little suspicious about why people might uncritically accept a medical definition of Alzheimer's as an appropriate starting point for its theological understanding. Medical definitions are helpful for medical proposes, but they may be considerably less helpful for working through the contribution of theology and pastoral care in the holistic process of defining and responding to Alzheimer's. Psychiatric medicine and theology can still communicate and cooperate around issues pertaining to Alzheimer's.

There is room for creative and critical discussion between the two (theology and medicine), but only if both are clear as to what it is that they are looking at. A classic example comes from Michael Ignatieff's book *Scare Tissue*, in which two sons are talking about their individual viewpoints regarding their mother's dementia and how they want to treat her. One son is a medical doctor and one is a lawyer.[60] Applying the principle, both theology and medicine must realize that two descriptions of the same thing may be both radically divergent and therapeutically similar. In order for this to happen, one needs a bigger story of Alzheimer's.

On a special note, two psychologists, Tom Kitwood from the U.K. and Steven Sabat from the U.S., have been deeply influential in providing the basis for such a counter-story for dementia and Alzheimer's. In different but deeply connected ways, they have challenged the standard story of dementia and offered important alternative ways of looking at, describing, and defining dementia. For them, dementia is as much *relational* and *social* as it is neurological. (see Chapter 8 and Appendix D for more about this subject).

2

From the Components of a Human to a New Creation of a Person

"So out of the ground the Lord God formed every animal of the field and every bird of the air, and brought to the man to see . . . and whatever the man called every living creature, that was its name." (Genesis 2:19, NRSV)

Thus far, the main problem for theology (medicine as well) is that the way in which one attempts to define and categorize Alzheimer's tends to result in a deep, component-like reduction of human persons. People are used to having their experiences of physical and psychological malfunction defined by others according to criteria that are general rather than specific to their situations. Rarely do they step back and wonder what it actually means to create and apply a generic term such as "dementia" to an unusual and deeply personal set of human experiences. Categorization is deeply interested in that which is general and universalizable, while theology and pastoral care are deeply interested in that which is particular and unique. The two positions are not necessarily exclusive of each other, but it is difficult for them to negotiate meaningfully with each other. The purpose of any process of categorization is to allow people to take elements such as ideas, and experiences, to observe their similarities and differences and, then to place them within particular schemes, the boundaries of which are marked according to perceived correspondences of kinds. The category of "dementia" thus indicates a particular form or configuration of relationships between personal experiences that are recognized and formalized in ways that allow for similarities to be noted, general explanations applied, and responsibility for care and intervention allocated.

A central part of the process of diagnosis and categorization is to break down the human person into constituent parts. Steven Sabat, who specialized in issues of the nature of the self within dementia, suggests that in the assessment and diagnosing of Alzheimer's, personal psychological life is made generic and broken down into certain components, such as the cognitive component, the intellectual component, the emotional component, and so on. These components are to be broken down into further "elements," such as memory, language, and function, and so on. Each of these elements is examined separately through the use of standardized tests in settings such as hospital clinics.[61]

Sabat also says that these components are measured according to the result of various psychological and neurological tests. Scores are then aggregated, and an overall picture of the person is constructed in comparison to a "typical dementia patient." The assumption is that dementia has a natural history that can be identified, tracked, and predicted, and which applies to all individuals who experience similar types of brain damage. The various tests that lead up to the diagnosis of Alzheimer's are designed to compare the experience and capacities of the individual to an average norm, then to assess and record the individual's current state on the bases of that norm. Once certain divergences from the norm have been identified, the task is then to establish the specific "cause" of the condition—that is, to track the linear cause-and-effect from the observation of particular experience, which are indicative of some form of brain damage, to the identification of the condition's formal cause. This in turn leads to some form of prediction about the future for all people with this condition, based on previous experiences of "typical" patients. This explanatory framework enables the doctor to understand the causes that lie behind an individual's manifest difficulties, irrespective of the particularities of their circumstances, and to look into and articulate the presumed nature of their future.

Such processes of causal determination, diagnosis, and prognosis are intended to capture and communicate the essence of the phenomenon of Alzheimer's. It is an epistemological and hermeneutical process intended to bring about clear understanding and accurate diagnoses leading to effective categorization and appropriate treatment. It is epistemological in that by configuring and naming a cluster of phenomenon or experience, it creates a new entity, which in turn provides new knowledge. It is hermeneutical in that the new entity becomes the primary interpretative principle that is used for interpreting the emerging situation and the continuing experiences of the person. In this sense, this process shapes a worldview. Breaking people down into their various components, renaming their experiences, and laying out the formal configuration of Alzheimer's in this way brings it into existence—medically and culturally—in quite a precise form. It is perceived to be a medical condition with distinct and universal features that are located specially or at least primarily within the human brain. Interestingly, at this point, Alzheimer's is a diagnosis by exclusion:

> It is what you have left when you have excluded all other sources of confused behavior. This is an impotent point. . . . Essentially it means that a diagnosis of Alzheimer's is often reached when the person doing the diagnosis cannot find any other explanation for the problems the person is experiencing.[62]

By this standard, dementia is inferred when other possibilities are ruled out. Through this process of exclusion, it is then presumed that people know what dementia is and what it is not. It is not temporary amnesia or delusion, it is not schizophrenia or bipolar disorder; by omission, it is not a social or spiritual disease. The one assumed certainty is that it is neurological through and through. Any emotional, spiritual, or social aspects are presumed to be epiphenomenal to the central neurological root. If such things are noticed or taken seriously, they must be read through the lens of neurological definition, which perceives them primarily as the product of failing neurology rather than as causal or explanatory aspects of the condition. It is suggested that the process of naming and categorization shapes a worldview. By reducing the core meaning of dementia to universalized typology, wholly contained within the biological, other potential core meanings and possible vital dimensions of the syndrome are excluded or at best downgraded. For example, forgetfulness is defined as a profoundly malfunctioning hypothalamus. Agitation is translated as a problem manifesting an underlying neurological pathology rather than a normal response to a frightening experience, or even an understandable response to the ways in which people have begun to treat the person with dementia. The person is assumed to have "deterioration in emotional control, social behavior, or motivation." The fact that such experiences might well be reasonable responses to a frightening life experience—conceivably resulting in a profound loss of memory—is lost in translation.

People's worldviews tend to be things they look *through* rather than look *at*. The subtle work carried out by definitions and diagnoses in the construction of worldviews often has latent malicious functions that are easily hidden beneath apparent manifest beneficence. Definition and categorizations are designed to provide people with maps that help them to make sense of certain experiences and objects in the world and to respond to them in effective ways. People easily misread these maps and fail to recognize that aspects of the terrain do not quite match up. The point is not that definitions and categorizations are in and of themselves unnecessary or dangerous. They may well be necessary, particularly for psychiatrists, for example, if less so for theologians. The point is that definitions and other ways of naming Alzheimer's are powerful storytellers that need to be recognized as such and challenged at the points where the story they seek to tell becomes misleading or erroneous.

Rethinking "the Obvious"

Take the core meaning of the name "dementia" in general (and Alzheimer's in particular), the literal meaning of which is "deprived of mind."[63] With this understanding, to have Alzheimer's is in some sense to lose one's mind. People do not have to look far before they come across this particular way of naming and defining Alzheimer's in both lay and professional language. Lawrence Broxmeyer makes this point quite nicely in his paper on Creutsfeldt-Jakob's syndrome: "Thinking and Unthinking: Alzheimer's, Creutzfeldt-Jakob, and Mad-Cow Disease: The Age-related Re-emergence of Virulent, Foodborne, Bovine Tuberculosis, or Losing Your Mind for the Sake of a Shake or Burger."[64] The tag line at the end draws attention to the issue at hand: *To have Alzheimer's is to lose one's mind.*

Even within popular Christian literature that genuinely seeks to advocate for people with Alzheimer's, the language of loss of mind can appear with benign intent but more malicious consequences. A book by Louise Morse about what it means for Christians to have dementia is titled, *Could It Be Dementia: Losing Your Mind Doesn't Mean Losing Your Soul.* It sounds like an innocuous, comforting title until the realization dawns about the underlying assumptions of Alzheimer's: First, it means losing your mind, and second, the soul is a place of God's redeeming activities that is separate from the mind. Both of these suggestions, as will become clear as the argument unfolds, are at the least open to question, if they are not in fact profoundly flawed.

Impaired Thinking

As mentioned, the impression that loss of mind is a central feature of dementia is not confined to lay definitions. As people have seen, the definitions of dementia by both the DSM[65] and WHO play into this way of thinking. Both in different ways claim that the syndrome people have named dementia includes impairments in *thinking* and *comprehension.* This assumption is presumably based on the types of tests that Sabat highlighted, designed to assess a person's cognition and comprehension. If one scores in particular ways on this particular test, one is assumed to have an impairment in thinking and comprehension. It makes sense, because people with Alzheimer's clearly do get confused, and certain cognitive tasks become difficult if not impossible. A significant problem arises, however, with global and unreflective ascriptions of *impaired* thinking. How do people know that a person's thinking is impaired? One can presume that thinking is impaired based on what is observed in the person's behavior, speech, or responses to certain questions on comprehension. The formal criteria, however, are behaviors, thinking and comprehension, and the latter can fluctuate based on variables such as mood, general interest, or the appropriateness of the subject matter of particular questions to the biography and personality of the individual. None of these factors are necessarily good gauges of what a person actually *thinks*. How does one determine that either behavior or linguistic response truly reflects what a person is thinking? Someone certainly can deduce that a person has impaired or changed behavior, or that their word choices seem to not make sense, or that they score badly on particular tests, but is it not much more questionable and presumptuous to suggest that one knows what others are *thinking*? Thought process are an aspect of the mind: they are not visible. They can only be presumed and inferred based on whatever criteria the observer chooses to use to interpret the person's behavior in any given situation.

Of course, it could be objected at this point that people actually do know more or less what others are thinking from what people see in their behavior. Wolfgang Kohler, a Gestalt psychologist, argues that "not only the so-called expressive movements but also the practical behavior of human beings is a good picture of their inner life, in many cases.[66] Kohlor notes that the process of understanding what is going on within the mind of another has less to do with mind-reading and inferring meaning from actions, and more to do with observing behavior without inference. If a person is startled by a loud noise, people do not infer the emotion of fear—they see it. People can see if someone is in pain, they do not infer the feeling of pain—they see it. If someone is upset because someone else asks them to do something, others see it rather than infer it from their actions.[67] People do not have to be mind-readers to understand a wide range of human experiences and emotions. Thus, it could be argued that it is quite legitimate to read thinking and distortion of thinking and comprehension into the behavior of people with advanced Alzheimer's. This brings up a crucial hermeneutical problem, however, because the reading of behavior is never done in a vacuum. People inevitably approach their subjects with particular theories, assumptions, and contexts in mind. In the case of Alzheimer's, too often they are too negative and too narrowly construed.

Confused Language

Beyond the issue of the hermeneutic of distance, the fragility of the statement that dementia has to do with impaired thinking is brought into sharp focus in a slightly different way in the work of Steven Sabat, who has shown quite clearly that linguistic confusion is not necessarily indicative of impaired thinking.[68] One may struggle for words or even use completely wrong words, but still be clear in what one is trying to say. The context and the person's own terms need to be heard rather than according to standard, preconceived normative assumptions.

Sabat highlights the fact that one should be careful with regard to the ways in which "impaired thinking" is tested. A person might be totally unclear in a test situation that focusses on what the researcher/tester considers to be significant, but utterly clear in other aspect of life that the researcher and those who construct tests are not interested in or do not see as significant. What people like this need is someone to take the time to listen carefully to them and to learn how best to interpret their "linguist confusion" and "impaired thinking." They need someone who has a map that is open to the type of terrain that they actually inhabit rather than a map that points out where they should be according to normative standards. They need someone to point out that they may actually be somewhere else, beyond the borders of the map, or that the map might be flawed or insufficiently detailed. If theologians or pastoral careers begin their approaches to dementia by uncritically buying into the assumption that they can somehow actually know that the person before them has "impaired thinking," the chances are that that is exactly what they will see. If, on the other hand, they are constantly prepared to give people the benefit of the doubt and leave open the possibility that what seems to be impaired thinking might in fact be communicating real meaning using a different map, surprising thing might happen.

Lost Mind (Mind-Less-Ness)

Perhaps the most poignant criticism of the suggestion that persons with dementia have lost or are losing their minds is the reductionist observation that no one really knows what is going on in anyone's mind other than their own. This is not an obscure philosophical point; rather, it is deeply practical observation. Jaber Gubrium, in his study of the social construction of the mind in people with Alzheimer's disease, presents a short but poignant abstract from an interview with a woman whose husband had the disease. In discussing the complexities involved in understanding her husband, the woman asks,

> How do you know his mind is gone? You don't real know for sure, do you? You don't really know if these little plagues and tangles are in there, do you? . . . How do I know that the poor man isn't hidden somewhere, behind all that confusion, trying to reach out and say, "I love you, Sara?"[69]

The woman was faced with quite a difficult dilemma. Which map should she follow as she is trying to negotiate her husband's tragic journey into Alzheimer's disease? She is well aware of the standard story of her husband's situation. She knows all about plagues and tangles and the medical narrative that speak of her husband's gradual decline and descent in to self-less-ness and apparent mind-less-ness. But like the philosopher's son's story, she does not feel she has to allow that story to be her only interpreter and guide on her journey. She chooses to take a different route and follow a different map and a different story.

How are people to understand this woman's statement? Either she is in denial and needs to be informed of the "reality" of her husband's situation, or she needs to be supported in her experience and affirmed that she may in fact be seeing different things than other people are seeing, and that what she is seeing may in fact be closer to reality. Denial is always a possibility, but, as Bogdan and Taylor's study has indicated,[70] so also is hidden insight.[71] In the end, like the philosopher's son, this woman chooses to give her husband the benefit of doubt. She does not abandon the medical story, but neither does she allow it to make her abandon her husband.

Out of (One's) Mind

The interesting way of drawing this point out is what people do when they visit a counselor or psychotherapist—*they tell them their stories*—in other words, clients give them the content of their minds. The professionals filter this content through whatever theoretical framework through which they have been trained to see the world. They then give them back their minds in a revised form, and if the clients do not agree, they are told they are in denial. That is a rather gross caricature, but it contains truth and helps to make the point. The mind is both an individual and a social/communal entity. Beyond the known mysteries, in whatever state it actually exists, then it certainly could be argued that it is the product of an individual neurology. But this is not the only place where the mind exists; it also has an existence outside of a person's individual body within the perceptions and presuppositions of the person's culture and those who surround them as those who read their minds into their actions and behaviors. Indeed, strange as it may initially seem, culture comes before mind. As Wittgenstein has ably shown, people have experiences first and then later develop thinking that reflects on those experiences.[72] The content of people's minds emerges from the language they use and the cultures within which they exist rather than the other way around.

As people learn language, they also learn that they have minds: as people engage with culture, the contents of their minds are shaped and formed.[73] Development of the mind is a second-order activity that emerges from community learning and living. In this sense, there is no such thing as "individual." People are deeply interconnected, even in those apparently private inner places typically ascribed to their minds.

That said, in order to make a statement such as "she has lost her mind," or even, "His thinking is impaired," people make three key assumptions: 1) They assume that they are competent to make such a judgment—but people are not, 2) people assume that the mind resides only within the boundaries of individuals' heads; again, it would appear that this is not in fact the case, and 3) people have a cultural tendency to assume that the mind is the essence of the person and that losing the ability to think clearly and intellectualize effectively is particularly important for who the person is and how his or her quality of life can be judged. Moving on, it will become clear that this also is not the case. On all three points, people could do better to give the demented person the benefit of doubt and see where that takes them. The overall point is that the suggestion that people with dementia lose their minds is highly questionable. Even if that were the case, it is debatable whether it would actually be possible for anyone to make that judgment. The very name dementia, meaning "deprived of mind," is a misnomer.

Going Beyond the Normal Story

How importance it is for theologians and pastoral careers to start their journey into dementia from the proper place? They have shown some of the problems that are tied up with the process of naming and defining dementia and have offered critical perspectives on commonly held assumptions about dementia that make all the difference in terms of getting to the correct destination. The point is not that theology cannot or should not converse creatively with the other disciplines involved in naming and caring for people with dementia. It is clear that such disciplines as psychology, neurology, and psychiatry contain much that is important and valuable to all parties concerned. The grounds on which to build that conversation, however, need to be established carefully and critically, and the territory inhibited by each discipline needs to be delineated and thought through. Spiritual experts have yet to develop the precise form of contribution that theology makes to the process of naming and redefining dementia. Suffice it to say for now that theology is not medicine, and the territory inhabited by medicine, while important for theology, is not definitive of either its starting point or its goal. From the perspective of theology, beginning the journey into dementia using the standard story as the primary map and guide will not take people to the right destination.

Categorizing and focusing on neurology to an extent are helpful for the mental health professions as they focus on pathology and treatment. But even here definition can be deceiving if their inherent and often hidden moral thrust is not recognized. The inner world of the person with dementia and those deep and intimate connections with the world outside are not inconsequential to what dementia is, and they cannot be narrated by neurology alone. Neurology may well keep telling about what has been lost, but as Ignatieff's philosopher's son knows, there is a need to keep telling the world that something remains. The story of what remains is a vital constituent of the definition of dementia that needs to be reclaimed. It is to the construction of such a story, which in this case is a *counter-story*, that the work now turns.

3

Question of Personhood

"First they came for the Jews, and I did not speak out because I was not a Jew. Then they came for the Communists, and I did not speak out because I was not a Communist. Then they came for the trade unionists, and I did not speak out because I was not a trade unionist. Then they came for me, and there was no one left to speak out for me."

—Pastor Martin Niemöler[74]

W hy might it not be such a good idea for "people" to be "persons"? Having begun to re-define Alzheimer's in fundamental ways, someone now needs to turn to a question that haunts many people: Is the person lost to the illness? How people answer that question will determine how they will respond to "persons with Alzheimer's." To answer such a question, one begins by exploring what it means to be a person in the first place, which is both complex and highly disputed. Within a culture that is marked by both hyper-cognition and hyper-memory (an excessive emphasis on intellect/cognition and memory), the temptation to define the nature of personhood and humanness according to such criteria is alluring and perhaps inevitable. Implicit within certain approaches to personhood is the assumption that in order to be a person (a person being something quite different from a human being), one must have certain capacities. Not to have these capacities is not to be a person, and not to be a person is to be excluded from certain moral and ethical rights and protections that are available only to those who are deemed to be persons. Primarily among such positive capacities that are presumed to comprise personhood are such things as intellect, cognition, memory, a sense of self over time, self-awareness, and an ability to value life. The potential problems that this way of understanding personhood might cause for people with Alzheimer's are obvious. By insisting that such attributes are central to what it means to be a person, such an approach implies quite plainly that, because people with Alzheimer's do not have such attributes or are losing them, they cannot be persons; thus, *to have Alzheimer's is to lose one's personhood.* Once again, an unsuitable conception takes a front seat in the perceptions of Alzheimer's, but this time the notion has slid into a moral quagmire—it has become a form of *moral imperfection.*

Better Dead Than Live

Unless the reader thinks that such debates about personhood are obscure and purely academic (in the sense of having no relevance for day-to-day practice), it is important to begin by noticing that while the discourse about personhood is formulated and conceptualized by academics in particular ways, it is actually quite a prominent feature in the daily lay conversations that surround Alzheimer's. It has previously been suggested that one of the ways in which people's understanding of Alzheimer's has been constructed is through a cluster of discourses, the dominant one being grounded in medical science. Within this interpretative framework, those affected are subsumed by their neurological condition, even to the point where they frequently are referred to as "dead."[75]

Previously, people have looked at the power of linguistic constructions to erringly position people with Alzheimer's. To linguistically construct people as imperfect is to place them within the parameters of those disciplines that are designed to seek out, fix, and mend that which is broken. To linguistically construct someone as somehow "not there" or not worthy of respect and attention is to allow the person's forgetfulness to become perceived and highlighted in society in negative and destructive ways. To linguistically construct people as *dead* is to position them in a way that inevitably evokes only responses appertaining to human death. A story will help draw out the importance of this point for people's understanding of personhood.

The Problem with Personhood

In order to understand how and why ideas of personhood have been formed and why they have a tendency to drift into maliciousness, people first need to examine the work that ideas about personhood is intended to do. At heart, philosophical models of personhood tend to be used as ethical devices designed to enable the separation of one group of human beings from the rest of humanity, normally in an attempt to assist practitioners or philosophers in working out how best to resolve specific dilemmas and deal with difficult ethical decisions. Those deemed persons are held under the banner of moral protection, and those deemed non-persons are not. So, for example, in the abortion debate, the justification for killing an unborn child is that the child is not a person, that it does not have certain capacities that would enable it to meet the criteria of any given definition of personhood. Thus, one is not killing a person but a "fetus"—that is, a non-person. This line of thinking can be dangerous for the cognitively disabled.

What Elements Comprise a Person

So what then is meant by the term "person"? To begin looking at this question, it is useful to start with John Locke's influential definition:

> a thinking intelligent Being that has reason and reflection, and can consider its self as its self, the same thinking in different times and places; which it does only by that consciousness which is inseparable from thinking, and as it seems to me essential to it.[76]

Thus, personhood here is defined in terms of a capacity for self-awareness, identity, continuity of thinking, a sense of self over time, consciousness, and above all, memory. Important for my purpose is the observation that memory is an absolute necessity for the other capacities to be possible. Noteworthy here is the inevitable way in which loss or absence of these capacities is accompanied by a loss of personhood. Viewed from this perspective, developing dementia means moving gradually and inevitably from personhood into non-personhood. This, of course, leaves people with the rather odd situation wherein certain human beings can be persons for sixty, seventy or eighty years, living out their final years (or days, depending on when the assessment is made about their personhood) as non-persons who gradually or suddenly become less worthy of moral attention and protection. The precariousness of such a position becomes clear when one considers that, in some ways, every time people fall asleep they become non-persons. Of course, it would be preposterous to justify killing simply because someone was not awake, but the slippery slope clearly is visible.

The Ethical Debate about Personhood and Dementia

From this perspective, it is easy to see how and why certain approaches to personhood make it look as if it would be just fine to euthanize people with dementia. Perhaps more than any other philosopher, the Australian ethicist Peter Singer has been at the forefront of challenging suggestions that people with profound cognitive disabilities such as dementia are persons. Singer also has become notorious for his views on the infanticide of disabled children.[77] In his view, to take the life of a severely cognitively disabled child is morally appropriate because such a child lacks the capacity for "self-awareness, self-control, a sense of the future, a sense of the past, the capacity to relate to others, concern for others, communication, and curiosity."[78] His indebtedness to Locke's definition is apparent, although precisely why "curiosity" should be an aspect of personhood seems more than a little arbitrary. Having said that, one should mention that curiosity *is* a trait that is highly valued by academics, which might explain why Singer values it about more obvious things such as love and relationships. Like Locke and Harris, Singer emphasizes the importance of consciousness and self-awareness and the importance of being able to value life:

> Only a person can want to go on living, or have plans for the future, because only a person can even understand the possibility of a future existence for herself or himself. This means that to end the lives of people, against their will, is different from ending the lives of beings who are not people. Indeed, strictly speaking, in the case of those who are not people, we cannot talk of ending their lives against or in accordance with their will, because they are not capable of having a will, on such a matter . . . Killing a person against her or his will is a much more serious wrong than killing a being that is not a person. If we want to put this in the language of rights, then it is reasonable to say that only a person has a right to life.[79]

Singer's understanding of personhood neatly excludes people with advanced dementia from the mainland of persons, leaving them stranded as if on an island, vulnerable, and well down in the inter-species hierarchy in terms of value and worth. The dangers of such malicious philosophical positioning are summed well by John Wyatt:

> Once this kind of definition is accepted, there are a number of logical implications. Firstly, it is immediately obvious that in order to be regarded as a person, you must have an advanced level of brain function. In fact, you must have a completely developed and normally functioning cerebral cortex. Secondly, there must be a significant group of human beings who are non-persons. These include fetuses, newborn babies, and infants who lack self-awareness, and a large group of children and adults with congenital brain abnormalities, severe

brain injury, dementia, and major psychiatric illnesses. Thirdly, there are many non-human beings on the planet who meet the criteria of persons. These include at least chimpanzees, gorillas, monkeys, and dolphins, but may also include dogs, pigs, and many other mammals. In fact, it has even been argued that within the foreseeable future some supercomputers may meet the criteria to be regarded as persons.[80]

From Singer's perspective, there is nothing unique about human beings. To suggest otherwise is to engage in "species-ism," a form of exclusionary practice that assumes human beings have some kind of inherent right to be perceived as more valuable that other sentient beings. The same criteria for personhood should be applied to all animals and not just humans. Once again, humans come up against the strange stress on the significance of the cerebral cortex. Researchers discussed the significance of the emphasis on the cerebral cortex when they looked at the way in which this aspect of the brain features in some key definitions of dementia. The idea that "higher cerebral functions" are important seems to be quite prevalent. One has to wonder what it is about this part of the brain that people seem to be so concerned about. Why should it be considered the biological seat of personhood, i.e., the neural correlate of the criteria that academics establish for what is and what is not a person? Is this not, as Wyatt suggests, a rather odd form of *cortextal-ism*:

In effect, Singer has replaced one form of discrimination with another. Instead of discriminating on the basis of species, he is now arguing that we should discriminate on the grounds of cortical function. In fact, if we are into name calling, we could call him a "corticalist." But why should corticalism be preferable to species-ism? Of course, Singer may wish to argue that cortical functioning is "ethically relevant," whereas species membership is not. But this is an arbitrary distinction that is hard to defend in entirely logical grounds. Why should the functioning of a 5mm layer of neurons be the central and only moral discriminating feature between beings? On purely logical grounds, species membership is a more coherent and fundamental basis for making ethical distinctions between beings.[81]

Wyatt's point is that a preferential option for a fully functioning cerebral cortex discriminates against people with mental impairments. There is a logical disjunction and a moral contradiction in replacing one form of discrimination with another. Why then might it be that academic philosophers like Singer choose contextually-oriented criteria to define persons and personhood? Wyatt uses the example of squirrels to illustrate that the criteria such philosophers use is arbitrary but understandable. If squirrels were in the position to choose which criteria might comprise special rights, they probably would choose agility and balance alongside the ability to eat nuts. Trees would focus on height or longevity. It is therefore not surprising that Singer, a human being with a fully functioning cerebral cortex who resides in a social context where the workings of this part of the brain are particularly prized, would choose to import his own values, abilities, and capacities into his understanding of what it means to be a person. It is likewise not surprising that he would exclude other things that are not important to him. The point is that the capacities that are said to comprise personhood are always worked out by those in positions of power; the powerless have nothing to say. The problem with capacities-based definitions of personhood is not only that they make certain people vulnerable to potentially deadly forces, but when looked at critically, they actually make little sense. "I am because I am curious" is an odd way to see the world. The arbitrariness of such criteria seems mystifying at first, but taking a closer look, one sees it is not mystifying at all, nor is it particularly subtle. Kitwood puts his finger on the issue:

Behind such debates a vague shadow can be discerned. It is that of the liberal academic of former times: kind, considerate, honest, fair, and above all else intellectual.

Emotion and feeling have only a minor part in this scheme of things; autonomy is given supremacy over relationship and commitment; passion has no place at all. Moreover, the problems seem to center on how to describe and explain, which already presupposes an existential stance of detachment.[82]

As long as Singer is healthy and cognitively functional, it is easy for him to dismiss those who are not, but what if Alzheimer's should visit him (or a loved one, as will be seen)?

The Problem with Egotism

Behind these types of debates about personhood lurks a particular view of what human beings are and should be and what desirable human living should look like. In other words, they are morally biased and deeply value-laden despite vain attempts to hide behind the mask of logical rationality. The particular worldview that underpins and drives the goals of Western liberal democracies has deeply shaped people's priorities and understandings of what is essential for their personhood. Within such a context, personhood tends to have a quite specific focus. To be a "person" means that one must be able to live one's life, develop one's potential, and develop a purposeful life course *without any necessary reference to others*. Importantly, the capacities that comprise people's constructions of personhood are not necessary for entry into the socio-political system, but they are considered necessary for a person to live in a way that can be deemed authentically human and thus valuable.[83] In this thinking, to lose the capacity to function in accepted ways is either to lose *something* of that which makes people human, or because it is assumed that humans are no more than the other animals, that which *actually* makes them persons. Within such a context, definitions of personhood that focus on self-awareness, reason, rationality, and so forth seem to make perfect sense. Warnock's comments indicate the inevitable outcome of such ways of thinking for people with dementia. The constructions of personhood that often guide people in their ethical and moral perceptions and decision-making are in fact prime examples of malicious social psychology. Likewise, they exemplify and give a philosophical rationale for the directly related type of malicious social positioning that Sabat has drawn to people's attention.

An Ethicist's Personal Experience with Dementia

One of the problems with the academic conversations about the lives of people with dementia—particularly advanced dementia wherein people lose the cognitive faculties that are the cultural markers of personhood—is that they do not work well in practice. It is one thing to sit in a classroom or a university office and pontificate about who is or is not a person; it is another thing altogether to act accordingly. Singer, as we have seen, is a strong and strident voice in the personhood debate and a firm advocate for the active euthanasia of people with severe intellectual disabilities and the assisted suicide of people with dementia. He retains this position consistently throughout his academic writings. In a hyper-cognitive culture, Singer's position seems to make sense—until, that is, the name changes from generic Alzheimer's disease to his mother, Cora, who was diagnosed with Alzheimer's disease. Within that subtle re-defining of Alzheimer's, things seem to change. Alzheimer's looks different when it has another name.

When Cora developed what was presumed to be Alzheimer's disease and was no longer able to recognize herself or her son (when she became a "non-person"), one would expect Singer to use her as an example of why euthanasia was a good thing and how awful it was that he was legally unable to put his writings into practice. One could guess that people might even expect him to kill her and accept the consequences of living out his own principles. His reaction, though, was quite the opposite, as his interview with Michael Specter in the *New Yorker* reveals:

> [Singer stated that he] would never kill his mother, even if
> he thought it was what she wanted. He told me [Specter]

that he believes in Jack Kevorkian's attempts to help
people die, but he also said that such a system works
only when a patient is still able to express her wishes.
Cora Singer never had that chance; like so many others,
she slipped too quickly into the vague region between
life and death.[84]

Singer's compromise is that, like Warnock, if Cora had had a chance
to leave a living will, then killing her might have been an option, but
since she was never able to do that, no one could know her wishes, and
so euthanasia was not an option. Interestingly, he begins his ethical
reflection by saying that he would never kill her before saying that it
would be justifiable in different circumstances. Why would he not kill
her? Presumably because he loved her? Love and pragmatic logic are not
always easy bedfellows, as Spector's interview revealed. When his mother
became too ill to live alone, Singer—instead of pressing the authorities
to allow her to die—hired a team of home health aides to look after her.
Spector asked him "how a man who has written that we ought to do
what is morally right without regard to proximity or family relationships
could possibly spend tens of thousands of dollars a year on private care
for his mother." Singer replied that it was "probably not the best use you
could make of my money. That is true. But it does provide employment
for a number of people who find something worthwhile in what they're
doing."[85] Specter recognized the moral basis for Singer's justification of
his response, but commented,

It hardly fits with Peter Singer's rules for living an ethical
life. He once told me that he has no respect for people
who donate funds for research on breast cancer or heart
disease in the hope that it might indirectly save them or
members of their family from illness, since they could be
using that money to save the lives of the poor. (That is not
charity," he said. "It's self interest.") Singer has responded
to his mother's illness the way most caring people would.

The irony is that his humane actions clash so profoundly with the chords of his utilitarian ethic.[86]

In the end, did Singer's experience with his mother change his perspective on his ethics of personhood? The answer seems to be yes and no:

> We were sitting in his living room one day, and the trolley traffic was noisy on the street outside his window. Singer has spent his career trying to lay down rules for human behavior which are divorced from emotion and intuition. His is a world that makes no provision for private aides to look after addled, dying old women. Yet he can't help himself. "I think this has made me see how the issues of someone with these kinds of problems are really very difficult," he said quietly. "Perhaps it is more difficult than I thought before, because it is different when it's your mother."[87]

As it happened, Singer's arbitrary assignment of personhood, which he readily applied to the less fortunate masses, suddenly became much more complicated with a diagnosis so close to home. He ended up caught in his own arbitrary net. "It is different when it's is your mother." Undeniably, it is, but it really should not have come as a surprise. Bernard Williams, quoted in Specter's article, puts it this way:

> You can't make these calculations and comparisons in real life. It's bluff . . . One of the reasons his approach is so popular is that it reduces all moral puzzlement to a formula. You remove puzzlement and conflict of values, and it's in the scientific spirit. People seem to think it will all add up, but it never does, because humans never do. Singer may be learning that.[88]

Calculation, comparisons, and neat formulas may make sense in a classroom or within the confines of a textbook, but when these decisions have faces, names, and consequences that touch people they know or those whom they have to touch physically and psychologically, things inevitably look different. Humans are much more complicated than rules and formulae can encompass. While people's scientific leanings may push them to make so-called rational decisions, one's personal relationships remain primal and inevitably draw them back from the unfeeling intellectual cliff when the closeness and intimacy of those relationships are in question. The language of capacities gives people distance and a perception of objectivity, but as soon as people are forced to come close, they learn that such language cannot really shield them from the deep pains of committed love. Coming close changes things.

Singer's "no" to change is manifested in the current update of his highly influential book *Practical Ethics*,[89] within which he, among other things, lays out the moral framework required to justify killing people with dementia. Unfortunately, his argument has not been changed or modified in response to his experience with his mother. It seems that sometimes people's reputation and history can take priority over what they really feel about a situation when it hits them in places where logic makes little sense.

It would be comforting to think that such arguments about personhood are extreme and that philosophers such as those examined here are unusual or unrepresentative; sadly, they are not. Anyone, it seems, can easily be tempted by models of personhood that, although often not articulated formally, are nonetheless powerful in their impact.

Relational Personhood and the Vanishing Self

> "Life is like an onion: You peel it off one layer at a time, and sometimes you weep."
>
> —Carl Sandburg[90]

Is there a person in "person-centered care"? Despite the problems with it, the language of persons and personhood remains a significant aspect of the ongoing discussion around Alzheimer's and its care. It could be argued that, despite the issues raised previously, ideas about personhood, given proper articulation, can and should retain an important place in the various conversations that go on around Alzheimer's. Such an argument has some validity. The types of person-centered models of care that have emerged from the kind of relational critique offered by Tom Kitwood, Steven Sabat, and others have—in some important ways—been among the most important innovations in the recent history of Alzheimer's care. A focus on the person as opposed to the label of "Alzheimer's" has offered fresh ways of trying to understand their experience. Nothing that has been said thus far should be read as taking away the significance of such person-centered approaches. Helping people to recognize the importance of coming close and recognizing the hidden possibilities within the person with Alzheimer's can only be a good thing. It may well be that the language of persons, properly articulated, should remain important; however, that really depends on what such language actually claims to represent.

There are three important issues that need to be raised regarding the ways in which the ideas around person-centered approaches to Alzheimer's currently are formulated. First, and perhaps in some ways most important, is the question about whether those working within the paradigm of person-centered approaches are actually using the term "person" in the ways that have been discussed. The language is similar, but is the conceptualization about persons per se, or does it have to do with developing particular attitudes toward people with Alzheimer's? In other words, is the term "person" only a container for ideas about the nature of loving care rather than a philosophical statement about the status of another human being?

Second, at a more philosophical level, underpinning the various person-centered approaches to dementia care is the idea that the root of all care and deep understanding lies in authentic personal relationships. Human beings are assumed to be persons-in-relation. Therefore, *good care is relational care*—to treat the other as a person is to relate properly and authentically with them. Inside this framework, the idea of personhood has come to be defined by relationships. If, however, to be a person is to be in right relationships with others—in other words, if persons are their relationships—then people with dementia have a significant problem. Most people do not want to be with them. If that is the case, many people with Alzheimer's *become non-persons by default,* even if personhood is judged according to relationality rather than capacities.

Third, and closely connected with the second point, it is not at all clear that contemporary Western liberal societies have the moral focus, desire, or strength required to create and maintain meaningful personal relationships with people who have significant cognitive and intellectual disabilities. Loving relationships and relational personhood require that people *choose* to be with people who have Alzheimer's. But why would they? In a social context marked by freedom, autonomy, and choice, the chances of anyone actually caring—other than those who feel obliged to care or who are paid to care—are not high.

Insofar as they focus attention on the uniqueness of individuals, person-centered approaches to Alzheimer's are exceedingly important. It is vital that those fundamentals that person-centered care represents remain a significant aspect of the territory of Alzheimer's and Alzheimer's care. Therefore, their position does need to be clarified, and the territory does need to be laid out clearly in order that theology can know its proper place.

The Person in Person-Centered Care

Let us begin with the first point: What kind of "person" does one find in contemporary understandings of person-centered care? David Edvardsson and colleagues sum the components of the person-centered approach, in which its proponents:

- regard personhood in people with Alzheimer's disease as increasingly concealed rather than lost;
- acknowledge the personhood of people with Alzheimer's disease in all aspects of care;
- personalize care and surroundings;
- offer shared decision-making;

- interpret behavior from the persons viewpoint; and
- prioritize the relationship to the same extent as the care tasks.[91]

This understanding of the goal of person-centered care is the embodiment of the type of values and revisions that emerge from the humanist-oriented theoretical thinking of people like Kitwood and Sabat and their relational understandings of Alzheimer's. Within person-centered approaches, the deeper philosophical claim that not to care in such ways means that the individual ceases to be a person is not normally expressed. The implication in much of the person-centered literature is not that there could be a situation wherein the individual could cease to be a person—only that it is important to value human beings. Therefore, the word "person" is not intended as a forensic tool or as an existential designator. Rather, it simply is a form of language that expresses a desire to value human beings and to care for them respectfully. Thus, Edvardsson, et al., can state,

> The rationale for the use of this concept is that "person," rather than "patient," is more consistent with the underlying humanistic philosophy of person-centered care for people with severe AD that is described in the published articles. Furthermore, the terms "person-centered care" and "good-quality care" are commonly used synonymously in the literature.[92]

The authors further indicate terms considered equivalent with "person-centered care": Various descriptions of person-centered care have been proposed, and concepts such as patient centeredness,[93] authentic consciousness,[94] skilled companionship,[95] senses framework,[96] and positive person work[97] are seemingly viewed as synonymous with person-centered care for people with severe AD.[98]

The term "person" is a designator for a general approach to caring for all people rather than a subsection of human beings. While the theoretical discourse outlined in the previous assumes that it is actually possible for people to become non-persons, the discourse around person-centered care emphasizes that to treat someone as a person is to treat them with value and give them worth irrespective of the presence or absence of particular capacities. The term "person-centered care" is a synonym for good care rather than a statement about someone's moral standing. One could substitute "valued and respected individual" for "person" without doing violence to the intention of the movement. Therefore, in an odd way, person-centered care in its secular humanist vein does not really need a person, at least not in the ways in which persons have been discussed thus far.

Relational Personhood

Nevertheless, despite the fact that there seems to be no formal articulation of models of personhood within many of the general approaches of person-centered Alzheimer's care, a more formal notion of personhood as a particular moral standing is part of the philosophical background of some key thinkers within this approach.[99] In exploring this, it will be helpful to return to the thinking of Tom Kitwood, behind which lies a formal notion of personhood. Within his approach, the antidote to malicious social psychology is positive personal relationships. Standing in sharp contrast, malicious social psychology constructs the personhood of individuals with Alzheimer's in particularly negative ways, while good personal relationships reconstruct their personhood in positive ways. Such a transition to the positive requires the particular understanding that *human beings are persons-in-relation*. Personhood is primarily a relational concept—it is not about one's capacities. The thing that makes a human being a person is one's relationships.

Persons are defined and held as persons in and through the relationships they have with others and that others have with them. The task of care providers is to learn to look at persons with Alzheimer's differently—as relational beings whose personhood is sustained in and through the relationships that people choose to have with them. When care-persons learn to look at people in this way, it will become possible to initiate a "new culture of care,"[100] which will stand in stark opposition to demento-genic cultures, [101] and in so doing will act as a brake on the types of malicious social psychology that, as people have seen, are so prevalent within society. This emphasis on relational personhood has been highly influential. It is certainly a significant and positive movement away from the types of capacities-based approaches to personhood that are so problematic for people with Alzheimer's. Care and caring relationships are what hold persons in their personhood, not their failing capacity to do certain things. At the same time, while the relational approach seems like a good place to begin to rethink the idea of personhood, there is one significant problem with this approach. If people's personhood is dependent on their relationships, what kind of relationships do people need to be sustained as persons, and what happens if they do not have them or cannot find them?

The Centrality of Relationships for Being a Person

In what is widely recognized as his most influential book, *Dementia Reconsidered: The Person Comes First*, Kitwood describes personhood as "a standing or status that is bestowed upon one human being by others, in the context of relationships and social being. It implies *recognition, respect,* and *trust*." [102] According to this understanding, personhood is not based on the presence or absence of particular capacities. Rather, it is a gift that is bestowed upon people by others, irrespective of their capabilities or capacities. Importantly, Kitwood suggests that the kind of relationships that counter malicious social psychology are *personal relationships*. If malicious relationships are marked by misunderstanding, devaluation, and mistrust, the personal relationships within Kitwood's model of personhood are marked by recognition, respect, value, and trust. Malicious social relationships move people away from the individual; relational personhood moves people toward them. The philosophical basis of this understanding of personhood lies within the thought of Martin Buber, who proposes that there are two types of human relationships: "I–It" and "I–Thou." [103]

"I–It" Relationships

To address another as an "it" requires coolness, conceptualization, detachment, and instrumentality. "I–It" relationships are analytical and conceptual; those within them are inclined to judge people and things according to their functions. Molly Haslam describes this relationship as a "bending back on oneself which develops into the attitude where the Other exists as a value-neutral object for the projects of the self."[104] The problem with I–It relationships is that they cannot reveal the wholeness of human beings. Such relationships are turned inward and determined by criteria other than the immediacy of the present moment of meeting. One cannot see another's whole being because,

> The otherness that is manifest in these relations is not that of the Other as Other but as the Other-for-me, and if the Other as Other cannot be wholly manifest here, neither can the wholeness of the self. The Other is manifest here as an object for the use of the self, as based on biological, sensorial, perspective, or intellectual functions of the self.[105]

"I–Thou" Relationships

When it comes to the lives of people with dementia, there is a tendency to treat them as "its" (an attitude that is deeply reinforced by the type of categorization that was highlighted previously) rather than "thous." Kitwood expresses it this way:

> Buber's starting point ... is different from that of Western individualism. He does not assume the existence of ready-made monads, and then inquire into their attributes. His central assertion is that relationship is primary; to be a person is to be addressed as Thou. There is no implication here that there are two different kinds of

objects in the world: Thous and Its. The difference lies in the manner of relating. Thus it is possible (and, sad to say, all too common) for one human being to engage with another in the I–It mode.[106]

For Buber, authentic human existence is encountered within the "I–Thou" relationship. To address the other as a "Thou" requires a non-objectifying moving toward the Other and into the space between one's self and the Other. In this space of meeting, one does not try to conceptualize or analyze the Other or to determine what it is that makes the Other different or otherwise. It is a place of true meeting. It is a movement toward Others that recognizes them as meaningful beings who are worthy of respect, people who are worth spending time with, sentient beings who are worthy of a certain kind of relationship.

Human—Person—[me-God] relationship

The reason that Kitwood would be drawn to such a perspective is obvious. As people with Alzheimer's begin to lose their capacities, it is the task of those around them to sustain and maintain their personhood by continuing to relate to them in particular ways, to see them and seek to be with them simply for who they are. As long as one is recognized as a person, one will remain a person. This is indeed a powerful counter both to the models of personhood discussed thus far and to the various practices of malicious social psychology and positioning encountered daily by people with Alzheimer's. The problem is that if people's relationships comprise their personhood, then presumably if they do not have such relationships, they are no longer persons. In other words, by holding on to the idea of "personhood" as a definable ethical concept, Kitwood creates the possibility that non-persons actually do exist, which makes it genuinely surprising that he insists on retaining the language of personhood. The humanistic values incorporated in ideas about recognition, respect, and trust would do the work for him without his having to move into the language of personhood. Moving from these principles into a formal model of personhood seems strangely out of line with the overall intentions of his project. Jan Dewing captures this point:

> Kitwood's conceptualization of a person can be located within personhood theories, albeit from a revisionist perspective. This, in effect, produces a major inconsistency that goes against what his work is trying to achieve, as personhood theories ultimately are about rejecting and excluding humans based on restrictive definitions of persons and the attributes required for being a person.[107]

If, as Kitwood suggests, personhood is a standing or status, then presumably some people are included and others are excluded; otherwise, there would be no need for the category of "person" in the first place. If that is the case, then Kitwood actually does not offer a counter-position to the personhood theories of people such as Locke, Harris, Warnock, and Singer; rather, he ends up simply confirming that they have a point. It is, in principle, possible to be human and not be a person—people with Alzheimer's really can and really do become non-persons in certain circumstances. If malicious social psychology is real and prevalent, then the possibility of many people with Alzheimer's actually being or becoming non-persons is a real concern. Knowing God and knowing one another are deeply interconnected. Since personal relationship with God are of the same basic nature as proper, authentic human relationships, then it follows that having a relationship with God contributes toward understanding the nature of proper, authentic human relationships. As people come to know God, as they experience God, they are enabled to know what it means to be in authentic relationship with others.

Therefore, there is a theological and an epistemological distinction that, as Stuart Charmé points out, is used to establish a parallel between relations with other people and relations with God.[108] This epistemological distinction is matched by an ethical distinction relating to how people should be treated.

God is a Person, and God's way of relating with human beings is deeply personal. People may not be able to know all that there is to know about God, but at a minimum they can know the basic form in which God chooses to relate to human beings—he relates personally. More than that, God is the "absolute Person,"[109] the person who first created humans and then became human, who defines human persons, and who cannot be limited:

> It is as the absolute Person that God enters into direct relation with us. As a Person, God gives personal life; he makes us as persons become capable of meeting with him and with one another. But no limitation can come upon him as the absolute person, either from us or from our relations with one another; the man who turns to him therefore need not turn away from any other *me–God* relation; he properly brings them to him, and lets them be fulfilled "in the face of God."[110]

God, the absolute Person, enters into personal relationships with human beings; this relational movement provides the shape and form of the personal and enables people to engage in "I–Thou" relations. It is as people encounter God in the space between and experience God's relational movement toward them that they come to know and understand what it means to enter into analogous "I–Thou" relations with others.

It is, however, important to be clear about how people might understand such terms as "relational movement" and "God's movement toward people." A crucial aspect of the I–Thou relationship is that it is a non-conceptual and non-mediated objectification of the Other. Nor does it require the mediation of the Other through any external systems of categorization. As soon as people try to work out exactly what the Other is or precisely what it is people are experiencing, they inevitably move into the me–others mode. When people do this, they "reduce the presence of the Other to the past as its uniqueness is considered only in terms of what it has in common with others people have encountered."[111] When Jonathan Franzen refers to his father's Alzheimer's disease as nothing more than as instance of what millions of other people are going through, he moves his father from God to an Other and allows that perception to mediate his encounters. People can be in the present moment with people with Alzheimer's only when they learn how to be with one another without mediation.

The "I–Thou" relationship is a place of experiencing without conceptualizing, of being without knowing. In this sense, there is indeed a deep apophaticism about the "me–God" relationship. What can one know about God? How can one conceptualize the divine? Thus, when people talk about recognizing God's relational movement toward them, they are not talking about rational, analytical knowledge. Rather, they are talking about experiencing God without having to name who God is and encountering another without having to name that Other. The "me–God" relationship in its human analogue has to do with experiencing and being with one another in the space between them, a place where people do not have to "know" who the Other is in order to really be with them, and they do not need to "know" them in order to be related to. For now, the key thing to notice is that the "me–God" relationship that requires them to conceptualize and recognize one another in cognitive ways.

It is clear, therefore, that the "me–God" relationship is not just an ethical relationship; it is deeply spiritual and profoundly theological in origin, meaning, and intent, revealing as it does some deep things about God and how God relates to human beings. To omit God from a person's understanding of persons is to misunderstand at a deep level the profundity and theological importance.

The "me–God" relationship is firmly rooted in God's movement toward human beings. It is not dependent on response, but it does shape the types of response that mirrors the divine approach. To be a person is to be in a "me–God" relationship specifically with God. People may be wary of the non-specificity of God and the depth of the apophaticism (denial) that his God seems to reside within. Nonetheless, the important point is that the security of human personhood is wholly determined by God—the absolute Person—who unchangingly reaches toward human beings in "me–God" relationships. Even if human beings do not or cannot respond, they remain persons as God the absolute Person continues to relate with them.

Here is the recognition that personhood has to do with God's desire to relate and that God's fashion of relating is personal. Such a position cannot be proven empirically, but *it can be shown by living it out*. One who engages in "me–God" relationships bears witness to a personal relationship that transcends one's own desire to relate. As people live out that reality in their personal relations with others, they bear witness to a different order, within which human beings are shaped and defined by "me–God" relationships, which begin with the divine and find an echo in the living witness of all embodied human beings.

4

Alzheimer's — In the Context of Creation

"What are human beings that you are mindful of them, mortals that you care for them?" (Psalm 8:4)

"The glory of human beings is not power, the power to control some-one else; the glory of human beings is the ability to let what is deepest within us grow."
—Jean Vanier, *Befriending The Stranger*[112]

Many of the stories told about and around Alzheimer's are both enlightening and troubling. The various stories told by medicine, psychiatry, psychology, neurobiology, and philosophy are all in some ways helpful and necessary in terms of developing a fuller understanding of Alzheimer's and facilitating good practice and authentic caring approaches. Likewise, it is important to be aware of relational and linguistic dimensions of Alzheimer's and how they function within social contexts, as well as practical theology and pastoral care perspectives, which have something to offer with a view to enabling a more faithful form of practice. Taken together, they can point toward the places where relational theology and spiritual care should begin their journey into Alzheimer's. An interdisciplinary approach to Alzheimer's is fully appropriate as long as each of the participants is read critically and none is allowed to define the whole of the terrain that Alzheimer's inhabits.

It was suggested that medicine, psychology, and the other disciplines that have been used to understand Alzheimer's and develop strategies for caring for people with Alzheimer's need to be recognized as practicing within the specific context of *creation*. The task of practical theology is not simply to reflect theologically on current understandings of the world of Alzheimer's; rather, it is to show the difference that it makes when people recognize that all that is known about Alzheimer's and Alzheimer's care emerges from a theological context. That context precedes and deeply shapes everyone's knowledge of Alzheimer's, and by which it is seen to be inherently theological, even though it often is not acknowledged as such. When people seek to define and understand Alzheimer's within the context of creation, that context makes a difference in every aspect of the disease.

When viewed within the perspective of creation, sin, and redemption—that is, from within the counter-story told in the strange new world of the Bible—Alzheimer's, like all of human experience, looks quite different. As people listen to this narrative and seek to respond to its redefinition, this powerful counter-story—the theological shape and intention of the journey into Alzheimer's—will become clear.

Personhood and Humanness

To unpack the implications of defining Alzheimer's and practicing Alzheimer's care within creation, it will be helpful to pick up on personhood and see what being a person might look like when it is defined from the perspective of the Christian story. Robert Spaemann makes an important argument against the idea that human beings are somehow defined by their capacities:

> Human beings have certain definite properties that license us to call them "person"; but it is not the properties we call person, but the human beings who possess the properties.[113]

- 48 -

From here, he means that there may be certain things that are associated with personal existence such as the ability to communicate, relate, respond, and so forth. These things might be considered aspects of persons, but they emerge from persons rather than being definitive of persons. In other words, being a person comes prior to any particular capacities that might be associated with personhood. As Spaemann affirms, "Recognizing a person is not merely a response to the presence of specific personal properties, because these properties only emerge where someone experiences attention which is paid to persons."[114] In other words, personhood precedes capacities.

Spaemenn further sees that personhood is not a genetic category that brings certain benefits to some people and prevents others from receiving them. He sees it as, "being a person is no more general category that the concept of 'person' could specify."[115] To be a person has to do with possessing *a way of being* rather than a set of capacities. This way of being perceives the material content of human (bodily) existence, not as the place where personhood is produced, but as the medium through which it is expressed and lived. Thus, personhood is seen to be situated within the life of human beings:

> Fundamental biological function are . . . specially personal performance and interaction. . . .They are embedded in rituals; they provide the focus of many forms of community life . . . the biological function is integrated in a personal context, often as the highest form of expression of a relation between persons. The kinship connections . . . are not merely a biological given, but personal relationships of a typical kind, relations which as a rule last for life. Human personality is not something over and above human animality. Human animality, rather, never was mere animality but the medium of personal realization. The nearer and more distant kinship relations in which human beings stand to one another are of personal and so of ethical, importance.[116]

Human existence is personal existence because it is always lived out within the human community—even that which is biological is personal. To be a person is to be a member of human race. Berndt Wannenwetsch summarizes Spaemann's approach on this point:

> Rather than being an instantiation of concept or a member of a class, a person is "but a participant in a community of mutual recognition." There is no "potential person" any more than there can be only the "idea" of a person." "Person" as a concept exists only as long as there are individual persons. If "person" is not a generic term but rather the way in which individuals of human genus exist . . . then "each of these individuals occupies an irreplaceable position in the community of persons, which we call mankind"—and it does so not by co-option but by birthright. "There can, and must, be one criterion for personality, and one only; and that is biological membership of the human race."[117]

To be a person is to be a member of the human race; it is to be born into and to participate in the human family. Such participation is not determined by any particular capacity or set of capacities, but rather by "genealogical relationship of kinship":

> Members of the species *homo sapiens* are not merely exemplars of a kind; they are kindred, who stand from the outset in a personal relation to one another. "Humanity," unlike "animality," is more than an abstract concept that identifies a category; it is the name of the concrete community of persons to which one belongs, not on the basis of certain precise properties objectively verified, but by a genealogical connection with the "human family." . . . Belonging to the human family cannot depend on empirically demonstrated properties. Either the human family is a community of persons from the

word go, or else the very concept of a person as "someone" in his or her own right is unknown or forgotten.[118]

Within the human community, the dual and unshakable premises of birthright and mutual recognition bind together all of its members. Membership of that community is biological and genealogical and therefore clear and irrevocable. There is no generic category of "persons"; being a person is a statement of particularity and participation in the human community. That being so, the ideas of "potential persons" or "non-persons" make no sense.

Spaemann moves away from personhood toward an understanding that insists that we value personhood rather than any particular properties that individual persons might contain. As members of the human race, all human beings are by definition persons. Personhood relates to the way that human beings are in the world and how they relate to one another and the world. It is not a set of capacities, and it is not simply a standing that is bestowed upon someone by others. It is an irrevocable status that comes from being a human being.

This understanding of the nature of personhood has much potential for people with Alzheimer's. There is nothing that can occur that can make someone less of a person. As long as one is a member of the human race, one remains a person who is valued and included within that genealogically interconnected family, bound together by shared birthright. Just as "Nothing can separate us from the love of God" (Romans 8:38–9), likewise, nothing can alter our human status as persons. Human beings are indeed persons-in-relation, and relationality is fundamental to personhood, which is not optional—it is an inevitable entailment of being human.

In Trinitarian terms, the theological significance of Spaemann's suggestion about relationality being fundamental to personhood becomes clear. Human relationality aligns in parallel with divine relationality.[119] The inherent relational nature of human beings emerges from the nature and relational shape of the God in whose image we are created, a God who is a Trinity of persons. God is a perichoretic community of love constituted by the relationships of three persons of the Trinity—God the Father, God the Son, and God the Holy Spirit—each one of whom is inextricably interlinked in an eternal community of loving relationship. Two points are noteworthy about the concept of perichoresis: 1) it indicates a coexistence of each member with the other that is marked by both distinction and complete unity or communion, and 2) it begins with the premise that each member of the Trinity is already a person, quite apart from their mutual relations.[120] There is of course no temporal sequence or separation between their being as persons and their being persons-in-relation, but the point remains apt. It is not the relationships among the Trinity—Father, Son, and Spirit—that make them persons; they already are persons. As they engage in mutual relationships of love, identity is bestowed upon each by and through the others. They all need each other in order to be what they comprise together. To bestow identity on one another, however, is not dissonant with them already being persons.

Something similar to this divine dynamic is apparent within human personhood. All human beings are irrevocably persons; to be human is to be a person. As human beings come together in community where they discover and develop their capacities and come to recognize themselves and become recognized as part of the extended human family. Human beings need one another to be who they are (Tom Kitwood). Recognition and identity formation are the tasks of the human community. When people are recognized as persons, authentic personal relationships become a real possibility, but even so, persons exist independently of their relations. They are *a priori* human beings who then form relationships. For this, the human family is an analogue of divine relationality—a community of persons who are called to be one family.[121] Viewed from a Trinitarian perspective, Spaemann opens up new possibilities for our understanding of personhood that overcomes some of the shortcomings in both capacities-based and relational models of persons.

The meaning of being a Human

For people with Alzheimer's, the question of being a person and a member of the human family pivots on the question of what it actually means to be human and what it means to belong to the genus *homo sapiens*. Evolutionists inform people that being human is simply the by-product of blind, natural forces working over time to produce other organism whose meaning and goal are simply to produce other organisms. Humanist argue that the term human is nothing more than a factual designator that indicates the value of people without any need for transcendence. Ethicists and philosophers tell people that they are simply a species among other species who have no particular moral claims over monkeys, pigs, or gorillas. Biblical creationists,[122] in contrast, argue that all things were created about 6,000 years ago and that human beings are the pinnacle of God's creation. Clearly, what it means to be a member of the biological category *homo sapiens* is most unclear. Yet, people need to be clear about what it might mean to claim to be human being and how that might relate to what it means to be a human being with Alzheimer's.

It is impossible to understand the full meaning of being a human person without first understanding who God is and where human beings stand in relation to God. Unless and until people begin to recognize and acknowledge the position of human beings before God, the situation of people with Alzheimer's cannot be fully understood, their personhood cannot be fully authenticated, and their care cannot be as effectively implemented. Without that understanding of what it means to be human in this light, we cannot begin to understand and live out the truth that to be a person is to be a participant in a community of mutual recognition and acceptance. Only in this context will we be able to maintain a proper focus on those aspects of what it means to be a human being that are most relevant to the questions raised by the experience of Alzheimer's.

What follows are a series of contextual meditations on humanness that emerge from contemplation on the experience of people with Alzheimer's that are relevant to the ways in which we understand humanness. In this way, the insights presented will contribute to the wide conversation on theological anthropology, while at the same time retain a specific focus on the human experience of Alzheimer's.

Embodiment: Breathing Life into the Earth

The first reflection on what it means to be human considers that people are creatures who are contingent beings, gifted with life and loved for who they are. Human beings are embodied creatures and cannot be reduced to their bodily functions, yet their bodies do matter. People experience the world in and through their bodies, without which it is difficult to imagine what it would look like to know God, feel and experience love, and engage in personal relationships. The bodied nature of being human also matters for a proper understanding of dementia.

Walter Brueggemann points out that contingency and embodiment are deeply interconnected:

> The human person is formed of earth and is breathed upon by God, to become a "living being" (*nephesh*). It means that the human person is, at origin and endlessly, dependent on the attentive giving of YHWH in order to have life. . . . The human person has vitality as a living, empowered agent and creature only in relation to the God who faithfully gives breath. Thus the human person is to be understood in relational and not essentialist terms.[123]

To be human is to be in relation with YHWH, our Creator:

> YHWH as creator of humankind and of each human person is sovereign in that relationship. Human persons are creatures who are dependent on YYWH and created for obedience to YHWH. Even before any concrete content is applied to the commands of YHWH and the obedience of human person, the category of sovereignty and obedience is a crucial and definitional mark of human beings.[124]

To be a person-in-relationship is a status that is promised, gifted, and sustained by YHWH the Creator. The relational nature of human beings is captured in the dynamic between the sovereignty of God and the obedience of God's creatures. Human beings' *natural* position is one of obedience under the security of God's sovereign power. Our *unnatural* position is one of disobedience and the autonomous exertion of human power, capacities, and desire.

Human beings are a strange combination of the material and the immaterial. Gilbert Meilaender quotes St. Augustine, who aptly described human beings as *tera animate*, "animated earth."[125] Genesis 2:7 talks about the way in which Adam was created:

> And the Lord God formed man of the dust of the ground, and breathed into his nostrils the breath of life, and man became a living soul. (KJV)

Human beings are thus created from matter; they are given breath and brought into living existence by the very breath (*nephesh*) of God. Matter understood without its necessary connection to that which transcends matter is misunderstood and misnamed. People are their bodies as they are their souls. The two are one; one cannot exist without the other.

Wendell Berry makes this observation:

> My mind has been deeply influenced by dualism, and I can see how dualistic minds deal with this verse (Gen. 2:7). They conclude that the formula for man making is: man = body + soul. But that conclusion cannot be derived, except by violence, from Genesis 2:7, which is not dualistic. Therefore, the formula there is soul=dust + breath. According to this verse, God did not make a body and put a soul into it. He formed man of dust; by breathing his breath into it, he made the dust live. The dust did not embody a soul. As it lived, it was a soul. The soul here refers to the whole creature. Humanity is thus present to us, in Adam, not as a creature of two

discrete parts temporarily glued together, but as a single mystery.[126]

The breath—*nephesh* in Hebrew—is "the vital principle of life itself, without which a person dies. . . . It refers to the animal essence of life with which every creature must endued.[127] The Hebrew word *nephesh* in English means "soul."[128] It does not relate to a discrete, immortal dimension of human person; rather, it refers to the in-breathing of God's Spirit into dust, which creates a living entity.[129]

Wheeler Robinson's phrase holds that a human being is perceived as "an animated body, and not an incarnated soul," a point that John A. T. Robinson helpfully develops:

> Man does not have a body; he is a body. He is flesh-animated by a soul conceived as a psycho-physical unity: "The body is the soul in its outward form." There is no suggestion that the soul is the essential personality, or the soul (*nephesh*) is immortal, whilst the flesh (*basar*) is mortal. The soul does not survive a man—it simply goes out, draining away with the blood."[130]

Without the life-giving *nephesh*, a creature cannot exist. Human beings are thus animated souls, or perhaps better, embodied souls, whose very breath and sustenance are wholly dependent on God for their continuing force, which is instilled within all creatures by the Creator God when he brings that which had no life into life. It is this *nephesh* that, as Glenn Weaver correctly point out, makes us connected with God at a deep level:

> The human *nephesh* . . . refers to continuing relationship of our identity to God. God's act did not plant some divine entity in a body which then gave persons a generic claim to eternal existence. *Nephesh* is not a divine form or force that humans have within. *Nephesh* is what happened when God brought into existence of any other

specific person, Adam. Adam's existence, and existence of any other specific person whom he represents, remains completely dependent on the moment-by-moment breath of God that upholds that life. As long as the breath is in us, we may live in responsibility and love with God. The description of Adam's walking before God in the Garden of Eden immediately follows the record of Adam's creation. It is likewise our "being" to walk with and to praise God."[131]

Human beings are animated earth who contains the very breath of God. As animated souls, one's *raison d'être* is to be with God. This is a critically important point. As earth animated by the breath of God, human beings are seen to be "holy creatures living among other holy creatures in a world that is holy," according to Wendell Berry.[132] Creation, therefore, is not independent of the Creator; rather, as Berry puts it,

> The human *"nephesh"* . . . refers to the continuous, constant participation of all creatures in the being of God. Elihu said to Job that if God [would] "gather unto himself his spirit and his breath, all flesh shall perish together." Creation is God's presence in creatures. The Greek Orthodox theologian Philip Sherrard has written that "Creation is nothing less than the manifestation of God's hidden being. Thus, we and all other creatures live by a sanctity that is inexpressibly intimate. To every creature the gift of life is a portion of the breath and spirit of God."[133]

If this is so, then attending to God's creatures is in fact a modem of attending to God. Jesus makes a similar point when he says, "I tell you the truth, whatever you did to one of the least of these brothers of mine, you did for me" (Matt. 25:40). There is something of God in all human beings[134] and something holy in all encounters between humans. The corollary of this, of course, is that depersonalizing God's creatures and treating them unjustly and malignantly positioning them is doing the same thing to God.

Relativization—A Fundamental to Personhood

Relationality has emerged quite prominently in the reflection on contingency and embodiment. At one level, human beings were created not much different from other creatures and shared common elements with them. At another level, however, being a human necessarily requires creatureliness.[135] What makes human beings different from the rest of creation is revealed in the sixth day experience of creation when God began to communicate with Adam and, for the first time, entered into a personal relationship with him. Genesis 1:28 highlights the unique offer of relationship that this relationship contains—extended only to human beings, not any other part of creation—on a personal level. This is not speciesism; it is an aspect of God's sovereignty and providential action toward the world he created. It is this dynamic, relational movement of God toward Adam that marks him out from the rest of creation. It is noteworthy that nothing internal to Adam makes him special, and God clearly is bound to and loves all of the creation to which he has given breath, but human beings are somehow different.

No explanation is given for God's choice to personally relate to humans. Absolutely none of this is Adam's doing—God initiates and God sustains the relationship. Even the catastrophe of the Fall and the relationally destructive power of human disobedience do not stop God from relating. It would have been better if Adam had done what God had told him to do; nonetheless, God's relational desire was not contingent on Adam's obedience or disobedience. It is Adam's status as a human being that is the sole criterion for the relationship that God chose for him. This divinely given gift of relationship is an inalienable source of human identity,[136] value, worth, and dignity.

In Genesis 2:18, God's relativization finds an important counterpart in the desire of human beings to relate to each other. Despite the fullness and goodness of creation, and God's gift of loving relationship toward

Adam, he was still incomplete. In response, God provided him with someone to whom he could relate and be with at a temporal level. The other creatures could not fulfill that function. Adam loved Eve, and only Eve, a fellow member of the human species who was both similar and dissimilar to himself, and who alone could fulfill his longing for human relationship. Thus Adam found his fulfillment[137] as a human being when God entered into personal relationship with him, after which Adam immersed himself in a personal relationship with Eve. Without God, Adam could not exist; without Eve, Adam was in some sense incomplete. With Eve and with God, he found fulfillment.[138]

To understand the theological significance of loneliness of people with dementia, human beings have a deep and primal craving for relationships with God and with others. There is no reason to suggest that this desire, which is common to all human beings, is not just as common in people with dementia. People with dementia find themselves caught up in malignant processes that threaten to destroy both their relationships with God and others. Not to have relationships is to enter a state that God clearly says is "not good." Thus, relational isolation on a temporal level is a deeply spiritual and theological matter.

Loving Relationships in All their Complexity

At the heart of human relativization is the desire to love and to be loved. To be human is to be loved; to live humanly is to love. Josef Pieper reflects on the nature of love in his book, *Faith, Hope, and Love*:

> In every conceivable case, love signifies much the same as approval. This is first of all to be taken in the literal sense of the world's root: loving someone or something means finding his "probus," the Latin word for "good." It is a way of turning to him or it and saying, "it's good that you exist; it is good that you are in this world!"[139]

Love is an act of engagement with another at a deep and personal level, which clearly states an inward action: "I want you to exist! Loving is therefore a mode of willing."[140] The love that Pieper focused on is not romantic love, which focuses on positive feelings, desires, and a longing to be with someone—Pieper's willful or intentional love is different. It requires determination, fidelity, and an intentional desire to be with the other and continue to love them no matter what. This is precisely the way in which God loves his creation, and it is precisely the way that human beings are called to love one another. The reason Jesus tells us to love our enemies is because not to love them is to behave in a way that is less than human. To hate the other is to suggest that we really wish that they did not exist—it is to act in a way that denies the reality of love and is a way to act inhumanly. This is why malicious social psychology is so dangerous. It not only dehumanizes people with dementia; it also dehumanizes those who engage with those with dementia. Thus, care for those with dementia that is truly person-centered in the ways described here is re-humanizing for all concerned.

Such intentional love is the kind of love one sees God showing to his creation. God brings creation into existence as a loving act of his will. He looks at it and at humans and says, "It's good that you exist; and you are in the world."[141] When creation rebels against God, his intentional love persists. When human beings become amnesic about their nature and their roots, when they live lives that are internally loveless, God persists. When God is disappointed by what is happening, his love still pushes forwards. To be human is to be loved persistently; to live humanly is to show persistent love toward others. Engaging in personal loving relationship is not the product of moral obligation or choice; it is a matter of faithfulness. Learning to love people with dementia—with all the issues, disappointments, hurts, and joys that accompany such a calling— brings into sharp focus one's vocation as a human being, which is to willfully and intentionally love one another as God has loved us: "A new command I give you: Love one another. As I have loved you, so you must love one another" (John 13:34).

As all people know, love inevitably is complicated, and it predictably becomes more complicated within the context of dementia, when personalities and behaviors can change and one's loved one can appear starkly different than they once did. When the person one claims to love has changed so much that we hardly recognize their behavior or personality, it raises fundamental issues about the nature and practice of love. Anastasia Scrutton explored this matter this way,

> There are . . . questions about there being a duty or command to love—is it really possible to choose to love? Or does the command to love just put a burden of guilt on to someone who is already suffering? And if we can't choose to love, what on earth are we doing when we make marriage vows? If it is possible to choose to love, aren't there situations in which it becomes more healthy and helpful to everyone involved to stop loving someone or to stop loving in a certain way?[142]

The point here with regard dementia is that as the condition continues, as a person's abilities to relate change and even seem to disappear, so the ways of understanding and practicing love inevitably will change. Nonetheless, these changed modes of love, as they work themselves out in the day-to-day routines of living with and sometimes struggling with people who have dementia, are no less authentic than the modes of love that one sees more often. They are just different. As a caregiver or family member bears witness to the changes and struggles to love the person in the way they did previously, it is necessary to recognize that love changes and the relationship changes. The point is to begin to reflect on what this "new love" looks like and to recognize the diverse and innovative ways in which one can say to the person with dementia, "It is good that you exist; it is good that you are in the world." Within the context of dementia, love might look quite different than it usually does; but love nonetheless remain love, even if it changes its shape in confusing ways. People's new tasks are to perceive, understand, and respond to the changes.

The Reality of Human Sin and Fall

Because the basis of creation is love in relationship with God and others, and the proper status of human beings is inevitably and thoroughly contingent on that premise, the tragedy of being human is the limited freedom given to them, which has challenged the potency of love. The creation story informs human beings that they are creatures loved by God beyond measure, creatures whom God considers to be "very good." The necessity remains, however, of recognizing one's contingent state within God-designed relationships and the centrality of their resonance in human's individualized and autonomy-driven cultures. In seeking autonomy, self-sovereignty, and God-like freedom and knowledge, human beings managed—and continue to manage—to alienate themselves from their one source of life and love, which is to reject the sustaining love of God. It is in rejecting the recognition of the absolute necessity of human obedience, dependency, and contingency that human beings find God's loving embrace toward them loosened—not because God loves them less, but because their desire to be loved becomes distracted by their desire to be free.

The importance of recognizing the fallen nature of the world for understanding dementia emerges from how one reads and understands the consequences of the Fall. The traditional Genesis account holds that human beings were created as immortal beings, who through the folly of the Fall, lost their immortality as the punishment inflicted on them by God. Thus, dementia can be perceived as a direct consequence of human disobedience and unnatural consequence of God's punishment. Another account of the Fall is that human beings were always mortal beings.[143] They were always dependent on their life-giving, *nephesh*-filled relationship with God. They may well have lived forever, but only as a consequence of God's sustaining breath. By choosing to turn away from their source of eternal sustenance, human beings encountered mortality, not as a potentiality, as it had been before, but now as a reality that impacted every aspect of their lives. Accordingly, the human race as a whole now finds itself living mortally in a world that has chosen to turn away from its primary relationship of love. That turning away and turning inward has consequences that are manifested throughout creation. *Thus, there is no direct connection between dementia and sin.*

However tragic, such a perspective on mortality is in a strange way helpful for the development of a positive understanding of dementia and how dementia sits within God's creation. To be human is to be mortal, and mortality means the decay is inevitable. Being so, our humanness is not diminished by dementia or any other condition. Such conditions are simply part of what it means to be human beings who are living out our lives in a creation that is broken but also is in the process of being redeemed. When people develop dementia, they do not move from being persons to non-persons. Theologically, the suggestion that dementia destroys personhood makes no sense. It is like saying that if one gets the flu, one will become a pencil, or a similar absurdity. Change and decay in all of its forms are part of what it means to be human. To be human in a world that is not yet redeemed is to grow old and to forget things; it is to develop diseases.

Dementia, Humanness, and Life in All its Fullness

It has been to suggested that nothing exists apart from God's desire for it to exist. Strangely, this includes dementia. Wendell Berry says,

> We will discover that God made not only the parts of Creation that we humans understand and approve, but all of it: "all things were made by him; and without him was not anything made that was made" (Jn. 1:3). And so we must credit God with the making of biting and dangerous beasts . . . That we may disapprove of these thing does not mean that God is in error, or that the creator ceded some of the work of Creation to Satan: it means that we are deficient in wholeness, harmony, and understanding—that is, we are "fallen."[144]

To take up Berry's point is not to suggest that God is indifferent to the suffering that dementia brings. It is, however, to emphasize that dementia has meaning. It is not punishment; it is not the work of the devil. It is a mystery that is firmly rooted in God's creative and redemptive actions in and for the world. It may not be understandable, and it may make ones angry, distressed, even outraged, but it is not without meaning. In this sense, people with dementia are part of the flux of fallen humanity, but their condition does not alter their meaningfulness or their lovableness. Put it poignantly, despite the fallen human condition, everything we have and everyone we know exists because of God and is deeply loved by God. It is important for people with dementia to know they are loved. It is true that practices of love that surround people with dementia are difficult and complex, but the fundamental truth remains irrevocable. Human beings are both wanted and loved irrespective of their physical or psychological condition. It is not any capacity within them that gives them value, nor is that value bestowed by those around them. Human beings' value and their identity are held and assured by the God who created them, who inspire them with God's *nephesh*, who sustains them in the power of the Holy Spirit, and who continues to offer the gift of life and relationship to all of humanity. It is this powerful counter-story that has the potential to provide a firm foundation for dementia care that is authentically person-centered and truly faithful.

5

What Health Changes Can be Expected with Normal Aging?

"They will still bear fruit in old age" (Psalm 92:14).

B y the year 2025, persons over age 65 or over in U.S. will increase by more than 100%, in Japan by 136%, and in Canada by 200%.[145] In Europe, the numbers will be 100 million in the year 2020.[146] Person now 65 can expect to live another 17.4 years; 75 another 11.1 years and 85 another 6.2 years in average.[147] One-half persons of age 65 and older have at least two chronic medical conditions.[148] 50% will die within ten years,[149] which can be determined from the physical changes that occur in the major organ systems of the body that are related to the mental aspects of change as persons grow older.[150] Two specific items will be addressed that are closely related to these statistics—physiological and brain changes.

Physiological Changes

Aging is not a single event but a process that begins at birth, ends at death, and occurs at different rates and in in different ways for all people, and no two people age exactly alike. Aging, in fact, is a completely individual process. Aging is a continuum. Our bodies change when we age, and our health status is the result of many factors, including genetic, behavior, lifestyle, and environmental.[151] As a result, it is impossible to describe anyone as "typically aging" or a "typical older adult." The stereotypical images of aging people with gray hair, wrinkled skin, stooped posture, cataracts, impaired hearing, and dementia, does not hold true. Such a picture is really a caricature of a typical old adult. Aging is more complex than that, and it occurs at different rates and in different ways. One person of the same age may be distinctly different from another in external appearance, behavior, and health. Recognizing that while similarities exist, there are individual differences that must be respected and treated accordingly. One's entire body does not age all at once or at the same rate. The assumption that all the organs in the body fail in concert is simply not true; people have different rates of organ decline. Chronological age tells little about the health of an older adult. Rather, functional age—what an older adult can do—is the more important indicator of health status of the older population. Their state of health may have a direct impact their emotional, psychological, social, and spiritual wellbeing.

There are many theories about why human age or grow old. Scientists believe that human bodies are programmed to age. This means that aging follows a biological timetable, possibly a continuation of the same timetable that controls childhood growth and development. Others believe that aging is due to damage to human body systems causing things to go wrong. There are two passages in Scripture that speak of the length of human life: Genesis 6:3, stating that "in the future" the human lifespan will not exceed 120 years, and Psalm 90:10 saying "seventy years are given to us."

Researchers do not agree about why or when humans age. Life expectancy (referring to the length of time that one can expect to live) and life span (the maximum length of life biologically possible for a given species) are interchangeable but mean different things. The life span of humans is believed to be about 100 to 120 years, with 122 years as the maximum. Undeniably, living longer is the result of advances in medicine and medical procedures, and doctors are able to help people fight diseases that once were considered life threatening. Genetics, environment, and lifestyle are three important factors in determining whether someone will lead a long and healthy life.

The Brain

The brain makes several changes during our lifetime as we go through the normal aging process:

- There is a small decrease in brain weight (smaller brain size) and increase in space between the brain and the skull.
- There is a gradual loss of brain cells, which are replaced at a rate of about 1% per year after age 60. Because of the tremendous reserve capacity of the brain, this loss of cell associated with normal aging has few noticeable consequences.
- There are also chemical changes in the brain with aging that may cause mild slowing of movement and somewhat Parkinson-like appearance in older adults—head bent forward, stiffening of posture, shorter steps.
- Three additional major afflictions affecting the brain in older adults may speed up and add to the changes of normal aging—1) Alzheimer's disease may affect 25% to 47% of person age 85 or older, 2) Parkinson's disease, and 3) Stroke—each of which affects 10% of those persons. As many as two-thirds of the brains of persons at age 85 or older have been affected by one of these three major afflictions.[152]

Changes in the brain with normal aging result in some decline in memory, which has been called "Age-Associated Memory Impairment." These memory changes are completely normal and expected. They do not progressively worsen or herald a disease process such as having trouble remembering a friend's name or why you went into a room, and so on. These same people do not have difficulty functioning in other aspects of their lives. They do not become confused or get lost driving in a familiar environment. They continue to perform complex tasks like balancing checkbooks, paying bills, scheduling and keeping appointments, preparing meals, and so forth. The memory changes associated with normal aging become more noticeable after a person reaches the age of 75 or 80. In fact, such memory changes do not worsen rapidly and will not interfere with a person's normal activities or relationships to any great degree.

Changes in brain function with age also results in older adults needing more time to learn new things, especially technology. Given adequate time, older adults can learn and retain information as well as younger persons. Understandably, older adults may need a little more time to remember and retrieve information from their memories, but often it comes to them normally. It is also worth mentioning that changes in the brain and nervous system with normal aging may cause some minor problems with balance, coordination, and reaction time. These normal changes may be worsened by disease or medications.

Understanding the Plastic Brain

According to Kitwood, the human brain events take place within a particular apparatus that has both structure and architecture:

> The key functioning part is a system of around ten thousand million . . . neurons, with their myriads of branches and connections, or synapses. A synapses is a point at which a "message" moves from one neuron to another, thus creating the possibility of very complex "circuits." So far as is known, the basic element of this system, some general features of its development, and most of the "deeper" forms of circuitry are genetically "given." On the other hand, the elaboration of the whole structure and particularly the cerebral cortex is unique to each individual and not pre-given. The elaboration, then, is epigenetic, subject to processes of learning that occur after the genes have had their say. Each human face is unique; so is each human brain.[153]

Unlike the other organs, such as the nervous system, the brain is plastic. Its shape, form, and development are responsive to and formed by the environment and the physical and psychological experiences that we have throughout our lifetime. From birth, the brain— unlike toenails or hair that grow to a predetermined genetic pattern—is shaped by experiences. What happens in the world around us—experiences, relationships, feelings, and so on—are all registered in and impact the developing neurology of our brains. "We are our experiences" is a profound way of describing the human brain.

To say the least, we can recognize the necessity of world 3 for development of the human person. The brain is built by genetic instructions (by nature) but development of human personhood is dependent on the world 3 environment (by nurture).[154] Neurologist John Eccles' key point remains pertinent: emotional and intellectual development and their neural correlates are essentially communal and physical from the earliest stages of infancy. For example, to develop a capacity to speak, one has to be spoken to, and for one's brain to develop effectively, one needs certain forms of relationship and experience. Relationships have neurological as well as psychological and social significance. The following were observed in dementia patients:

First, their brain structures varied significantly, not only according to their genetic endowments, but also according to the levels of learning and the types of experiences that they had. Kitwood puts it this way:

> Neuroscience now suggests that there may be very great differences between human beings in the degree to which nerve architecture has developed as a result of learning and experience. It follows that individuals may vary considerably in the extent to which they are able to withstand processes in the brain that destroy synapses, and hence in their resistance to dementia.[155]

Thus, resilience will differ from person to person.

Second, and consequently, there may be a much closer correlation between the experience of dementia and neurological damage that a person experiences. In other words, It may be that one's social experiences in some sense reinforce or perhaps even cause or exacerbate neurological damage and deterioration, which originally may have stemmed from different causes.

The Problem of the Mind-Brain Connection

In the heart of Kitwood's understanding, an implicit dualism is at work within biomedical understandings of dementia. His intention is to move people's thinking about dementia away from a Cartesian separation of the body from the mind and toward a monistic position that assumes the human being is a single complex organism within which there is no ontological or substantial separation between the mind and the body. Mind and body cannot be separate; thus the neurology cannot be understood without reference to other dimensions of human persons and their experiences. To focus simple on the neurobiology of dementia and ignore the significance of the mind is to misunderstand what dementia is and what its cause might actually be.

Kitwood's basic assumption and understanding of neurology, psychology, and social relationships is that "any psychological event (such as walking) or state (such as feeling hungry) is also a brain event or state and not psychological experience . . . causing brain activity . . . or vice versa; it is simply that some aspect of the rue reality is being described in two different ways."[156] Every psychological experience is at the same time a neurological experience and vice versa; the two simply represent two descriptions of the same event. Psychology and neurology are thus seen to be inseparably interlocked.

What is also important to notice is Kitwood's basic assumption, which is that "any mental state is also a brain event or state, instantiated in a brain with such-and-such a structure, which is the consequence of both developmental and pathological factors."[157] Two points are noteworthy: 1) there is a close tie between the mind and the brain; a person's experience leaves a physical mark on their neurology, and 2) mental states and brain events take place within a discrete brain that has developed in unique and particular ways according to the types of experiences encountered during life. Therefore, some persons are less likely to succumb to the types of brain damage that form the syndrome of dementia because of the ways in which their brains have been structured through their experiences over time.[158]

No two brains are the same or respond in the same way to neurological trauma that initiates the process of dementia—some are more vulnerable to the effects of brain damage and others are more resilient.[159] There is no such thing as a "typical dementia patient"; even if people at one level share similar forms of brain damage, it does not make them the same.

While dementia clearly relates to neurological damage and change, the actual impact of certain damage will be variable and personal. This is why some people have quite extensive brain damage but do not manifest dementia, while others with relatively little damage do exhibit the features of dementia. Kitwood's perspective suggests that the causal direction of neurological damage may not be straightforward. It may be that *events experienced outside of the body can actually impact what is going on inside the brain.* Therefore, we need to find out why the brain comes to develop the structures it does in the way that it does.

Spirituality and the Brain

Our brain in terms of our spiritual life remains quite fundamental. Is it not the case that many if not all of the things that we associate with spirituality and knowledge of God relate to experiences that clearly have neural correlates?[160] If those parts of the brain are damaged, one's perception of spirituality and the things normally used to actualize one's spirituality are inevitably damaged. Does this not indicate that while embodiment might be important, the brain remains more important than other parts of the body? Our spiritual lives—that is, how we experience God and the things that we use to enable communication with God—are clearly impacted by the state of our neurology. Robert Davis, a Presbyterian minister who had dementia, gives a sense of what this might feel like in his autobiography, *My Journey into Alzheimer's Disease:*

My spiritual life was still most miserable. I could not read the Bible. I could not pray as I wanted because my emotions were dead and cut-off. There was no feedback from God the Holy Spirit. As I tried to fall asleep, only blackness and misery came, misery so terrifying that I could not drop off to sleep. Night time was horrible. My mind could not rest and grow calm but instead raced relentlessly, thinking dreadful thoughts of despair. Invariably I lay there, terrified by a darkness that I could not understand.[161]

"Failing neurology can impact feelings of spirituality and the normal spiritual practice that we use to establish and stabilize our spiritual lives," says Davis. There is no denying that damage to the brain has serious consequences in this regard. Ray Anderson notices the centrality of neurology for manifestation of spirituality, saying,

Physicality sets limits to our personal existence and, at the same time, produces the phenomena we recognize as manifestations of the soul. In other words, there is no manifestation of the soul that is not produced through the brain even though the brain is not the sole effective cause. Therefore, we should not be surprised and should indeed expect that the firing of selective brain cells affects what we might call spiritual impulses, attitudes, and actions.[162]

The use of the term "soul," not in a dualistic sense, but rather as a descriptor of those aspects of spiritual life such as prayer, faith, and hope that normally are attributed to the soul. The point is that an embodied soul, as Anderson noted, is deeply influenced by its biological capacities, even when it comes to those impulses and actions that we have come to call spiritual. Reading scripture, remembering passages, meditation, prayer, and so on—all these things require our bodies and, in particular, our brains to be functioning in specific ways. Malfunctions in our neurology inevitably will have a deep impact on what we previously considered to be central to our spiritual lives. At a creaturely level, we should not be surprised that many of the traditional manifestations of the soul have neurological correlates that are deeply impacted by the degenerative processes of dementia. Part of being human has to do with the fragility and neurological dependency of our spiritual lives. Since we are embodied souls, it could be no other way.

Losing spiritual practices and experiences is not indicative of God's abandonment. He is always with us as long as he continues to sustain us through his *nephesh*. As long as we are alive, God's *nephesh*—our fundamental source of spiritual dynamism—remains (the significance of Steven Sabat's Self 1). Dementia cannot de-spiritualize people because God is Spirit, and unless God withdraws his Spirit from us, spirituality remains (spirituality understood in terms of our connectedness with God). In those who are experiencing dementia, spirituality may take a different form than it did before, but it does not disappear along with some vanishing neurons. Someone's inherent holiness is not affected by neurological decline, even if their previous modes of articulating it change or become unavailable. The challenge is for those around people with Alzheimer's to explore how best this holiness can be sustained in the midst of profound changes.

Spiritual Identity

The key to is to recognize that our spiritual lives, not to mention our very existence, are contingent and dependent. Contemporary approaches to spirituality have a tendency to focus on the actualization of the self as the primary criterion of authentic spirituality. If spirituality is self-actualization, and if the spiritual self no longer has the capacity for standard ways of developing, then failing neurology inevitably will be equated with failing spirituality. The essence of true Christian spirituality, however, is not self-actualization. At the heart of a genuinely Christian spirituality is God's approach to human beings—his *nephesh* brings us into existence and sustains us in that existence. The Holy Spirit comes to us in the midst of that existence and acts to sustain our spiritual existence quite apart from our ability to articulate that experience. It is the Spirit who sustains us in our spirituality and in our identity.[163] On the issue of human identity and how it is affected by the inevitability of bodily change over time, Anderson reflects that

> spiritual self-identity, as used theologically and on biblical grounds, is contingent upon the spirit of God both as its formation and its growth. The existence of brain cells is a necessary but insufficient condition for the expression of the life of the soul as personal spiritual beings.[164]

Brain function clearly is an aspect of our spiritual development and identity formation, but our identity is wholly contingent on the movement of the Spirit, who is the sustainer (Ps. 104:30, NRSV). Anderson presses us toward an understanding of human identity as something that is both given and sustained by the Holy Spirit.[165] The Spirit forms and names the living soul, the *nephesh*-inspired body. The brain plays a part in this process of human development, but it is not definitive or determinative. It is God the Holy Spirit who determines who a person is; the brain as an aspect of the body simply participates in the movement of a person toward that given goal. We do not actualize ourselves; rather, in some sense or another it appears that we are told who we are.

Self-identity, like the entirety of human existence, is wholly and radically contingent. Although at one level, neurology may be central for the aspect of experiencing our spiritual lives, at another level both our neurology and our spiritual lives inevitably are contingent on the Spirit of God. Anderson puts it this way:

> In a Christian anthropology, human nature is not defined ultimately by tracing humanity back to its origins. Or by explaining humanity in terms of its existence under the conditions of sin. Rather human nature is life experience as a personal body/soul unity, inspired and empowered

by the Spirit of God. Self-identity is both determined by the Spirit of God within each person and acquitted by the person through experience and interaction with the physical, social, and spiritual environment. One could say that each person has an identity that is more or less dependent upon the subjective life of the self, as well as at an identity that is projected upon from and by the Spirit of God. Even in our mother's womb, the psalmist says (Psalm 19:13–16), we are given personal identity by God.[166]

Therefore, human beings are seen to have an internal identity that is deeply influenced by our physiology and our social experiences, as well as a divine identity that is projected upon us in and through the Spirit of God. While both of these aspects are significant, they are not equal. Physiology and socialization are fragile, uncertain, and contingent; divine identity is given and eternally sustained. Human neurology, then, does not contain all that is necessary for the complete outworking of the life of our embodied souls. As Wendell Berry articulates, "we and all other creatures live by a sanctity that is inexpressibly intimate. To every creature the gift of life is a portion of the breath and spirit of God."[167]

This perspective pushes people to recognize the significance of the active present of the Holy Spirit at work in human beings, using but transcending the natural, creaturely possibilities of bodily existence. In Psalm 139:13–16, we are given into the work of the Spirit in both our formation and sustenance. It is God through the Spirit who knit together and forms all human beings. It is God who places the boundaries on our physical capacities. It is God who sustains and guides the whole of our lives. We are all limited, but even our limits have providential significance. Thus, our identity—who we *really* are—is envisioned, created, and held by God. Accordingly, there is a significant dimension of what and who human beings are that is not determine by our neurological or biographical history. This dimension is created, sustained, and nurtured by the Spirit of God quite apart from any particular capacities that we may or may not have. In this way, we can see that there is something eternal and given within all human beings that is wholly contingent on the Spirit of God. This eternal, Spirit-given dimension of human beings cannot be understood apart from its embodiment, and its eternality cannot be grasped apart from God's work of sustaining and redeeming.

It is through the body of Christ that human beings find reconciliation and redemption (Ephesians 1:7, NIV). Our bodies matter, because it is through the body that the gospel is proclaimed, prisoners are visited, the sick are consoled, and love is given hands and feet and voice. It is through the body that dualisms is broken down and meaningful care is practiced. It is though our bodies that we are able to receive others even when our abilities to articulate that experience have faded. As we care for bodies, so we care for souls. As Mary Jo Iozzio watched her mother care for her father, she noticed,

> How when we tend in particular to the bodily needs of another, we demonstrate a very deep respect for the person and faithful care for the material in which a person lives, and moves, and has being. . . . Care of another body challenges the intellectualizing tendency of dualism and elevation of spirit over matter. Any loss of bodily or mental control does not, by itself, remove or reduce the intrinsic dignity abiding in my father or everyone else.[168]

Bodies matter, and caring for bodies is as important as caring for minds. It is true that Cartesian predictions may make such a statement that feels counter-intuitive, but that is simply indicative of someone's enculturation in a particular, dualistic way of seeing persons.

The Heart and Physical Endurance

As people grow older, their heart muscles get stiffer, and they do not pump as much blood with each contraction. Their heart rates do not increase as when they were younger to compensate for a drop in blood pressure or to adjust to exciting situations. Even so, when absent from diseases, they do not cause any significant problems for any individuals such as weakness, loss of energy, or tiredness, all of which are all treatable. While physical endurance (prolonged physical activity) may decline slightly, it does not do so to a great extent as long as the older person maintains physical activity and keeps in shape. The heart has a tremendous reserve capacity that is never used. The reserve may be decreased as people age, but there is still more than enough left to enable older persons, even some extraordinary ones, to perform the usual tasks of living.

Skin, Muscles, and the Skeletal System

Because of reduction in fatty tissue immediately under the skin, the skin becomes thinner with age. It is more easily subject to tearing and bruising, especially on the arms and hands, because the skin is thinner and more susceptible to even mild trauma. Bruising may even be worsened by the regular use of aspirin or another medication for arthritis and other problems.

There is an increase in total body fat and reduction of muscle mass with age. Fat and fibrous tissue begin to replace muscle tissue, especially if muscles are not exercised. Again, however, because of the body's tremendous reserve capacity, these muscle changes cause few observable effects on strength or endurance, especially if muscles are used regularly. That can also be translated to, "If you don't use it, you'll lose it."

Changes also occur in the skeletal system with normal aging. There is a tendency for bones to become less dense and more brittle. This is especially true for women who have gone through menopause because the hormone estrogen helps to keep calcium in the bones. It is encouraged for women who have undergone an early menopause to receive estrogen replacement therapy. Osteoporosis disease—when too much calcium is lost from bones—causes the bones to become weak and fracture more easily, even with mild trauma. The hunched of over posture also caused by osteoporosis disease of many women is due to compression fractures of some bones that make up the spinal column.

Regular exercise, supplemental use of calcium, and estrogen therapy for some women can help to stem osteoporosis. Conversely, the negative side effects for estrogen therapy can be uterine and breast cancer.

The Internal Organs

Changes in the gastrointestinal tract, liver, and kidney are commonly associated with aging. One's ability to absorb food is slightly reduced, and function of the colon slows down, predisposing older adults to constipation. Prescription or over the counter medication may easily worsen normal changes from aging and result in some significant digestive problems (constipation, heartburn, ulcers, and so forth). Changes in the liver may affect the body's handling of medications. Most drugs are broken down or changed into their active forms in the liver. With aging, there is a reduction of blood flow to the liver, a decrease in its size, and a decrease in its capacity to break down drugs and substances. Liver damage caused by disease or alcohol can interfere with an older person's ability to tolerate certain medications, especially if the person is taking several different drugs, all of which are handled by the liver. The levels of certain medications can build up to become toxic. When prescribed for older adults, the doses of most medications should be reduced. This is particularly true for drugs affecting the brain and nervous system, the effects to which some may be extra sensitive.

Likewise, kidney function changes with normal aging and interfere with an older person's ability to rid the body of drugs that are eliminated by this route. Blood flow to the kidneys is reduced, making it necessary to prescribe lower dosages that must be excreted by the kidneys. They work together with the liver to expel drugs or other substances ingested into the body. This makes older adults more vulnerable to overmedication because the body cannot break down these chemicals in the liver and/or excrete them out of body through the kidneys as well as when they were younger.

Hearing and Vision

Normal aging brings some decline in hearing and vision. Hearing loss is usually more prominent for higher pitched sounds than lower ones. For this reason, older adults may be able to hear and understand deeper male voices better than higher pitched female voices. To make out sounds and words can be more difficult, especially on the phone, in crowded rooms, or in other noisy environments. Many diseases and toxic effects from certain medications can add to normal declines in hearing, producing problems that may seriously interfere with communication. These hearing changes can be corrected by hearing aids, and today's digital, programmed versions are significantly improved over previous analogue versions, but they can be considerably expensive for older adults (I speak from experience).

Changes in vision also occur with normal aging. The lens of the eye changes in composition, often requiring the use of corrective glasses or a new prescription to compensate. For this reason, regular exams by an optometrist are required. Difficulty with visual acuity only compounds difficulties with balance, depth perception, and judgment of distance, which can lead to falls and traffic accidents. Several afflictions affect the eyes in later life, such as cataracts (dimming and haziness), diabetes, stroke, and disease of the lining at the back of the eye—macular degeneration, which can lead to blindness. One in three Americans over age 75 have this disease and the numbers are projected to double from 11 to 22 million by 2050.

Psychological and Social Changes

Most persons experience little change in their personality or interests as they grow older. Persons who were outgoing and social (extrovert) when they were young or middle-aged likely will continue to be so as they get older. Likewise, those who were introverts or social recluses at a younger age also tend to retain these traits in their older years. In some cases, personality traits actually become more accentuated with age. In any case, older adults usually continue to enjoy the same things they enjoyed when were younger, which applies to work interests, hobbies, recreational activities, family, and even sexual activity.

Depression, sadness, loss of interest, or unusual withdrawal from social interactions do not occur with normal aging. These are symptoms of treatable maladies common in later life, which also includes sleep disturbances. As persons grow older, they normally experience a reduction in deep sleep and have more frequent awakenings during the night. Older adults also experience sleep phase advancement—both going to bed early and waking up early. Nonetheless, older adults need as much as sleep as young adults to keep them feeling energetic. Insomnia, hypersomnia, and apnea are common, treatable conditions in later life. If not treated, however, these issues may lead to emotional and physical health problems such as depression, high blood pressure, heart disease, and many others.

The American Geriatrics Society's *Complete Guide to Aging and Health* (Williams 1995) section on "How We Age" provides a wealth of practical information about physical and mental changes that occur with aging. The section, "Conditions that Affect Older People," explains the different medical conditions that elders commonly experience and discusses how to differentiate normal aging from these conditions.

6

Understanding Dementia

"This trail of unraveled brain structure and mounting dysfunction is, in physical terms, only one of inches yet its silent, implacable wrecking creates entirely new conditions for living life and being with others."
—Arthur Kleinman, *Caregiving: The Soul of Care*[169]

The term dementia (Latin, "out of mind") is used to describe a group of symptoms, a syndrome characterized by multiple cognitive and functional deficits of sufficient severity to interfere with daily activities and social relationships.[170] The loss of functioning in dementia is due to the death of brain cells, which can be caused by a variety of diseases. While some can be treatable or reversible, the nonreversible like Alzheimer's disease predominate in the geriatric (old age) population. Although progressive, the course of dementia symptoms varies depending on underlying disease processes. Dementia can mean different things for different people; it may express itself in many ways according to its diverse effects upon various individuals. It may even be that further research will indicate what we call "dementia" is an umbrella term that turns out to have diverse pathological processes. Currently, Alzheimer's is the leading memory loss disease among many types of dementia.

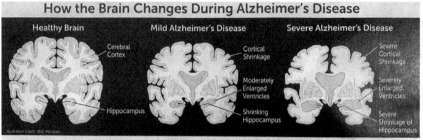

As Alzheimer's disease progresses, brain tissue shrinks. As the ventricles enlarge and the cells of the shrinking hippocampus degenerate, memory declines. When the disease spreads throughout the cerebral cortex, language, judgment, behavior, and bodily functions decline along with memory until death, usually 8 to 10 years after diagnosis. *Research is our only hope. Please give generously today.*

The causes of Alzheimer's disease are not known for certain, but hereditary factors play a big role in cases where the disease is genetically transmitted. More than 30 million people worldwide suffer from Alzheimer's disease—the most common form of dementia. The combined term dementia/Alzheimer's (or senility) indicates progressive, marked decline in intellectual or cognitive functions associated with damage to brain tissue, which may affect personality and behavior, and it may be of a reversible or irreversible type. In the aging process, once there is loss of memory, the immediate popular judgment is, alas, that it must be the onset of the dreaded brain disease Alzheimer's, which leaves the body still alive after the brain is dying or dead. We may call this a neuropathic ideology, reflecting people's scientific culture in which thought is more valued than love.

Alzheimer's disease is the most frequent cause (60% to 70%) of dementia. It is a brain and neurological disease and it is progressive. It occurs at increasing frequency with age (5% to 10% in persons over age 65 increases to 47% of persons 85 or older), amounting to almost half the elderly population. Alzheimer's disease is the fourth-leading cause of death in adults, after heart disease, cancer, and stroke.

The onset of the disorder is gradual, insidious, and characterized by declines in:

- Memory—losing objects, repeating stories, missing appointments, learning new information with difficulty,
- Language—difficulty finding the right word when speaking and when naming objects, advancing in the final stages to unintelligible speech and muteness,
- Visuospatial skills—difficulty cooking, setting the table, fixing or manipulating information in the home,
- Cognition—difficulty handling and manipulating information, performing calculations, making rational judgments,
- Personality—increased fatigue, indifference, impulsiveness, irritability, self-centeredness, and social withdrawal.

But we still are not certain that the above are real symptoms of Alzheimer's disease?

Alzheimer's disease is a clinical diagnosis; in other words, there is no practical test that can be done to definitively establish the diagnosis. Brain biopsy and postmodern autopsy are the only way to make a definite diagnosis of Alzheimer's disease. In its early stages, it is difficult to distinguish patients with Alzheimer's disease from those with "age-associated memory impairment" or "cognitive impairment" from other causes (multiple strokes, chronic alcoholism, brain tumor, delirium, vitamin deficiencies, thyroid deficiencies, syphilis the brain AIDS-dementia, et al.). The diagnosis is made by identifying characteristic pathology in brain cells. Most of the time, physicians make a presumptive diagnosis of Alzheimer's disease based on history from the patient and family, an examination of the patient's memory and other higher brain functions, and certain laboratory tests. In approximately 20% to 25% of cases, the physicians' presumptive diagnosis is proved wrong and some other cause of the patient's symptoms is found at autopsy. It is difficult to establish a diagnosis of Alzheimer's disease after a single evaluation; repeated mental status examinations every six months usually help to clarify the picture. A comparison and diagnostic history are always helpful.

The greatest cost of dementia, more specifically Alzheimer's disease, is not financial, even though its cost has surpassed the cost of treatment of cancer, heart disease, and stroke, it is more personal. This cruel ailment steals people's memories, steal people's independence, and finally steal people's dignity by eroding the ability to manage the basic tasks of daily life. As the population grows older, the number of Alzheimer's cases will continue to increase if we find no way to stop the disease.

Dementia, inclusive of Alzheimer's, can affect anyone of any age, unfortunately even children. Children diagnosed with the condition (childhood Alzheimer's, the degenerative effects on the brain) at a young age do not survive to adulthood.[171] According to the Alzheimer's Association, 5.2 million American had Alzheimer's disease in 2014. Nearly two thirds of sufferers are women. Dementia is a collective term for several conditions (see Appendix I) marked by a loss of mental abilities.

Generally, the disease begins near the hippocampus, the brain memory center, and then spreads to areas of the brain that control language, judgment, and physical activity. The disease was named after a German physician, Alois Alzheimer, who presented a case study in 1906. A build-up of proteins in the brain, the hallmark of the disease, forms clumps known as "plaques," which appear to contribute to the neuron death, and "tangles" of protein fiber that disrupt the neuron's transit system. Eventually, communication between neurons breaks down. It is degenerative, which is to say that the plaques and tangles get worse over time. There is no cure *but treatment appears to stop its spread in the brain.* There has never been a patient who has recovered from this disease.

Alzheimer's disease *is a physical process. It is not a mental illness.* Nonetheless, there may be mental/emotional problems attached, but *the illness is purely physical.* Experts emphasize that severe decline in mental capacity caused by Alzheimer's is not a normal (natural condition) sign of aging, but it is related to age. Signs of a clinical state of Alzheimer's disease (damage to the brain cells) are much more serious.

Since Alzheimer's progresses slowly, the disease can linger for years or even decades. Alzheimer's disease costs the U.S. some $214 billion annually, according to federal estimates. Generally, there is a stigma attached to Alzheimer's and other dementias; there is a great shame associated with Alzheimer's, especially for people with early-onset Alzheimer's. People think that when someone has Alzheimer's they disappear. Honestly, that is not the case—they are still present and still the same person—like the movie, *Still Alice*,[172] about a woman who has early onset Alzheimer's, portrayed by actress Julienne Moore.

Higher Cortical Functions

Before people move on to explore how they might go about redefining Alzheimer's disease, there is one farther observation that will be helpful. The ICD-10 definition of Alzheimer's disease is "a syndrome due to disease of the brain, usually of a chronic or progressive nature, in which there is disturbance of multiple higher cortical functions, including memory, thinking, orientation, comprehension, calculation, learning capability, language and judgment." Part of this definition, "impaired thinking," has been looked at, and it is open to challenge and reinterpretation. There is, however, another aspect that is highly problematic and deeply pertinent for people experiencing Alzheimer's disease within Western cultures in particular. This aspect relates to how this kind of definition emphasizes the significance of the "higher cortical function." This emphasis is also apparent in the DSM-IV's highlighting of disturbances of higher cortical functions as significant for defining the parameters of Alzheimer's disease. The definition is clearly intended to suggest objectivity, scientific rigor, and technical accuracy. Higher than what? When using of the spatial metaphor of higher cortical function? The lower ones, presumably, but why are these particular capacities considered higher? This point is more than mere semantics. Stanley Jacobson and Elliot Marcus describe higher cortical functions this way:

> What is a higher cortical function? As one examines the abilities of a human, one is struck our ability to use tool and create wonderful buildings or works of art. However, our ability to communicate by speaking and writing and reading, *"we believe,"* is the best example of a higher cortical function.[173]

The expression "we believe" in this statement is worthy of note. Higher cortical functions seem to be higher because they allow humans to do things that other animals cannot do—in particular to speak, write, and read. The author of the ICD-10 definition considers "higher" functions to be "memory, thinking, orientation . . . language and judgement. But why? What makes such capacities higher than the capacities to love, relate, touch, and feel—all aspects of experience that people with Alzheimer's disease hold onto throughout their journey? Why are capacities like orientation and comprehension higher than the capacity to weep and feel distress for the loss of those things that remain valuable but seem distant in the midst of profound memory loss?

The use of the term "higher cortical functions" implies that this aspect of the brain, the cerebral cortex, came into existence late in the evolutionary process, and that its functions are advanced in comparison to other aspects of the brain, which have not developed as fully or as with as much complexity as this part. Why call this aspect of the brain's development "higher"? Surely the essence of the theory of evolution—human beings are consciously or intentionally advancing from a state of primitiveness toward a state of higher consciousness, awareness, and capability. The argument of why this is so is a process of random mutations and genetic changes that occur over limitless periods of time—genetic formations, traits, and configurations that enhance functional effectiveness and enable adaptation and survival. In this sense, human brains are no higher or lower than they were at the beginning of the evolutionary process: there is nothing to progress toward or away from. Human beings cannot move upward or downward; they just move on. The spatial language of "higher cortical functioning" must at best be metaphorical, but what is the metaphor about? Is it coincidental that the capacities that are highlighted as emerging from the area of the brain that produce the "higher cortical functions" are precisely the capacities that are highly valued by contemporary Western societies? More precisely, capacities such as memory, thinking, language, and judgment are the aspects of human beings that are deeply prized by intellectuals, academic, and academic researchers—the very people who construct such definitions. In other words, this aspect of the definition is clearly culturally bound and value-laden. This observation about the emphasis on the cerebral cortex will become important in discussion of personhood. Here people must note that to indicate that acquiring Alzheimer's disease includes losing their higher cortical functions is a much deeper and altogether more alarming statement than it might at first appear to be. Hidden in the midst of this apparently objective and scientific statement is the subliminal suggestion that people with dementia are losing those aspects of being human which are perceived as more important than the other capacities humans might have. The truth is they are losing only that which society prizes the most. Receiving such a diagnosis puts people in a tricky position that has both neurological and social implications. Definitions are not value neutral; often, they are value-forming.

The Stages of Frontotemporal Dementia (FTD)

James M. Ellison, MD, MPH, Geriatric Psychiatrist at Swank Memory Care Center, Christiana Care Health System, focuses his current research on new medications for the treatment of Alzheimer's disease, and on lifestyle factors that affect the development of cognitive impairment in later life. Ellison also has received several awards for his teaching and other activities, including most recently the Massachusetts Psychiatric Society's 2014 Advancement of the Profession Award.

FTD is the diagnosis for about five percent of people with major neurocognitive disorders (dementia). About 70% of cases begin before age 65, so it is a more common dementia among the "young old." FTD involves degeneration of the frontal and temporal lobes of the brain. The frontal lobes are important regulators of behavior and the temporal lobes assist in our understanding and expression of language. The symptoms of FTD, therefore, include major changes in behavior, impairment of language, or both.

People diagnosed with FTD and family members often ask, "What stage of dementia is occurring?" and the answer to this question can be useful in knowing what to expect in the future. FTD often begins during the years when adults expect to be healthy and productive. The average course of the disease takes six to eight years after diagnosis, so patients and their families must confront serious and increasingly difficult needs. Detailed and complex timelines of the stages of FTD are not entirely accurate, but it is useful to think of the development of FTD through early, middle, and late stages. Let us look at the stages of frontotemporal dementias to see how these related disorders evolve.

Early-Stage Frontotemporal Dementia

It is in the early stage of FTD that each syndrome shows its most unique features. Memory is often spared at the beginning, and perhaps for this reason early stage FTD can easily be overlooked or misdiagnosed as a psychiatric condition.

The behavioral type of FTD, called *behavioral variant FTD*, affects social and personal behavior early on. Like a patient named Joseph, a person with behavioral variant FTD can start to disregard the usual social boundaries and say or do inappropriate things. They can behave impulsively, carelessly, or even criminally. Judgment and handling of money may deteriorate. Apathy is common and the person loses interest in hobbies and self-care. Empathy or concern for others' feelings and needs often diminishes.

The language-affecting types of FTD come in two varieties, paired together as *primary progressive aphasia:*

> *Semantic variant primary progressive aphasia*, in the early stage, is characterized by loss of names for people, places and objects, word-finding difficulties, and difficulty understanding specific single words. As in one patient's case named Barbara, grammar may remain correct despite trouble grasping the meaning of specific words. Behavioral changes are common, too, including irritability, trouble sleeping, depression, and emotional withdrawal. Selective eating and compulsive behaviors can develop.[174]

Non-fluent variant primary progressive aphasia, on the other hand, shows itself through the development of labored and halting speech, like another patient named Lloyd. Grammar is misused and speech sounds can be distorted. Patients are able to understand single words and simple sentences but get confused with more complicated sentences such as "The dog that belonged to Billy was running away."

Middle-Stage Fronto/Temporal Dementia

In its later phases, the symptoms of FTD variants become more similar and FTD also looks more similar to other dementias such as Alzheimer's disease. In behavioral variant FTD, people are likely to need more assistance with basic daily tasks, the so-called "activities of daily living" (ADL), such as dressing, bathing, and grooming. Disturbances of behavior become more frequent and consistent. Those whose problems initially were more behavioral can develop language difficulties and those whose language was more impaired early can develop behavior problems.

Late-Stage Frontotemporal Dementia

In the late stage, people with FTD look more similar to those whose dementia is due to Alzheimer's disease. Both language and behavior are affected and memory deterioration often occurs as well. It may be necessary to have care 24 hours per day to assure safety and adequate care. Death may eventually occur as a result of infections such as pneumonia.

As yet, FTD has no specific medication or treatment, but there are valuable information resources for caregivers and patients through the Association for Frontotemporal Dementia (AFTD). The behavioral symptoms of FTD sometimes respond to off-label medications to help with apathy, depression, mania, agitation, irritability, aggression, or delusions. Cognitive rehabilitation and speech therapy may address some language difficulties. Many researchers are seeking the understand the genetics, pathophysiology, and potential treatments for FTD, in the hope that research eventually will identify disease-modifying or preventive treatments.

In sum, I do not want to diminish the real pain and anguish that dementia can bring with it to the imperfect view of dementia. However, to define it in purely negative and sorely neurological terms is tempting but inappropriate. In fact, some of the central losses that are associated with dementia have been picked up and reframed to reveal either that they do not exist, or that if they do, they exist in a form quite different than "normal" assumptions suggest. Some of the corrections to assumptions follow:

- Dementia has to do with more than neurology and neurological decline. It is a complex psycho-social-neurological disease that has significant linguistic and relational component.
- Dementia is not something that is internal to an individual's neurological makeup. Dementia belongs to and emerges from some kind of community.
- Dementia does not entail a loss of mind. Rather, it provokes others to presume that there is a loss of mind. To suggest a loss of mind is to misunderstand the person in fundamental ways.
- Dementia does not entail a loss of self. The self remains intact even in the most severe forms of dementia. Any loss of self relates to a failure of community.
- Dementia symptoms such as aggression, depression, withdrawal, anxiety, and deterioration in emotional control, social behavior, or motivation may not in fact be caused by failing neurological process alone. When understood correctly, they can be seen as reasonable responses to difficult, frightening, and frustrating situations.

If such a person's situation is misunderstood and misrepresented, if he or she is treated according to what is presumed to be happening rather than what is actually happening, then communication breaks down and the possibility of a negative hermeneutic emerging between those seeking to care and those receiving care becomes a real possibility. This is not to suggest that damaged neurological functioning is not a significant aspect of the process of dementia. Its role in the process of creating dementia is not as central as it at first appear to be. Neurological function remains a significant inhabitant of the territory of dementia, but other perspectives are now beginning to reclaim some of the territory that has been lost. If ones takes these insights seriously and is prepared to give people with dementia the benefit of doubt, dementia begins to look different, and one's options for positive care are expanded. Seeing things properly makes a significant difference.

In order to understand the experience of dementia, ones need to first to understand the person's story. When one grasps both the disease and the story, the true structure and nature of dementia begins to emerge. This is not to suggest that dementia can be cured through relationships. It is, however, to put neuropathology in its proper place, and to draw attention to the deep and formative significance of the environment, the relationships, and the attitudes and values that surround a person who has been given the name of dementia. Such an understanding provides a firm and appropriate place to begin to reflect on the theological and pastoral dimensions of dementia, and the proper place to begin the journey is becoming clear.

7

The Necessity for
Redescribing Dementia

L ike any journey, traveling toward an understanding of dementia
requires starting at the right place with right tools: appropriate
route, maps, and transportation. Without those means, we will not reach
the right place where we intended to arrive. In fact, following the wrong
road map, we surely will end up in the wrong place. If we understood
dementia like this, in the end we will not know what dementia is because
we will not really have visited it.

Dementia is a multifaceted condition, and prioritized (culturally or
medically) a single facet and assuming it to be definitive of the whole
explanation is an unwise theological and pastoral move. Therefore,
a revised map of the territory of dementia is required to suggest that
theologians and pastoral caregivers might be wise to start their journey
in a different place from where they might "naturally" assume they should
begin. That place might seem strange and abnormal, but the journey
into dementia will reveal important new territories that will bring fresh
understanding and revelation.

Two Ways of Looking at Dementia

Michael Ignatieff's book, *Scare Tissue*, is a powerful and moving
semibiographical account of two sons' experiences with their mother's

development of Alzheimer's disease and her eventual untimely death.[175] It tracks the complex emotions that the family goes through as they wrestle with the difficult issues that emerge from watching and being with someone who is forgetting all that once made her the person they remembered and loved. It is a somewhat disturbing but beautiful reflection on the nature of self and processes that serve to "self" and "unself" people experiencing advanced dementia. At the heart of the story are two quite different sons (one is a philosopher, and one is medical doctor of the hard-nosed scientist type) and two quite different relationships with their mother. That book offers two ways of looking at dementia that result in two sharply contrasting stories that can be told about it.

The story pivots around the sons' shared experience of their mother's dementia and the distinctly different ways in which they each deal with it. The philosopher son narrates the world in terms of ideas, emotions, and alternative possibilities using sources of knowledge and inquiry. For him, it is the experience of dementia—both his and his mother's that is of paramount importance. The scientist son inhabits a story that perceives the world primarily in objective and empirical terms. This story is only about hard, cold facts without mystery or wonder. For him, what is true about dementia is that which is empirically provable and evidentially the case. This brother resides in a world where the scientific method and the technology that emerges from it reign supreme. It is perhaps not inconsequential that while he desires to know a great deal about the etiology and prognosis of his mother's illness, he rarely visits her.

In their now primary roles as caregivers to a person with dementia, both brothers see her quite differently. The doctor sees dementia as a medical entity that requires the marshalling of all the technical resources available in order to do battle with the condition that is destroying his mother. In contrast, the philosopher son's experience with his mother's dementia is deeply personal and relational, and he is wrapped up in the day-to-day life with his mother, refusing to abandon to negative external assessments of the disease. He knows that what dementia is cannot be separated from who his mother is and is becoming. He visits his mother every day.

Giving the Benefit of the Doubt

Unlike his brother, the philosopher son chooses not to accept uncritically the stories told about his mother by the professionals he encounters. His mother's true self has not gone; the mother he loved is not gradually disappearing. She is not losing herself as some assume. Because he knows her and what he sees when he comes close, *he wants to give her the benefit of doubt.*

Both look at the same person, but both see radically different things at the root level. They are looking at the same person but seeing her totally differently. One sees disease and disintegration and names it with technical terms; the other see his mother with all that such recognition implies. The latter son's task of positively recognizing and remembering his mother is a different one. The apparent obviousness of the cause of her dementia and the clear meaning of her neurological decline do not lend themselves easily to a different interpretation of her experiences, particularly when the naming power within the conversation is clearly to the advantage of the specialist—dementia is best understood in terms of damaged neurons.

Ignatieff's narrative of the two brothers' experiences of their mother's dementia illustrates well the difficult tension between the standard story of dementia, with its focus on the specifics of neurological decline and technological intervention, and the "hidden" story, which from the former view, sounds ridiculous and is easy silenced by the skillful use of technical language. And yet, the experience of the philosopher son tells us some deep things about the nature of the disease, even if his language and experience do not correlate well with the medical account. In order to understand why there is often such a disjunction and a tension between medical perspectives and the lived experiences of dementia, one needs to spend some time reflecting on how the concept of dementia came into existence in the first place and why the process of naming particular human experiences like dementia might be more complicated and deceptive than it first appears.

Naming Dementia—a Question of Definition

The criteria used by health care professionals to define exactly how dementia has been collated, simulated, and laid out in quite specific ways. Richard Cheston and Michael Bender note the following:

> At present two important systems of classifying psychiatric illnesses exist. The WHO sponsored the development, in 1948, of the ICD;[176] in the U.S. a slightly different system emerged known as the *American Psychiatric Association Diagnostic and Statistical Manual* (DSM).[177] Both of these systems have gone through many variations, with some illnesses being abandoned, others brought into being, and most altered, some radically. The latest versions are ICD-10 and DSM-5.[178]

These diagnostic criteria represent formal attempts to try to bring together and make sense of a variety of different human experiences—which experiences have been perceived as problematic by the people who have them, as well as their families and society. The specific collation and grouping of these experiences from the diagnostic criteria comprises an apparent consensus of practicing professionals. Although based on scientific research and observation, the process of defining and naming what are and what are not the constituent parts of dementia is not an objective process. The difficult history of the development of such criteria indicates that there is often little consensus among doctors concerning what should or should not be included within any given form of categorization. In other words, definitions always emerge from a context of contention and sometimes widely differing opinions. This is not to suggest that the general approach is not scientific. It is, however, to point out that the politics that surround the ways in which scientific data is worked with in this context is not objective or value free. Warren Kinghorn puts this point well in his reflections on the origin and purpose of the DSM criteria:

> The truth is that the DSM, like any psychiatric diagnostic classification, has never been an "objective" document in this sense. It has always been a pragmatic tool of a particular clinical community—starting with American psychiatric and extending, in recent years, to global psychiatry, to the non-psychiatric mental health professions, and to medicine as a whole—useful for fostering inter-clinical communication, for providing an operational base for the organization or research, for self-regulating and discipline in diagnostic practices, and for proposing to the public that particular states of affairs are best interpreted within the language-game of psychiatry.[179]

Kinghorn highlights the important point that classificatory systems such as the DSM or the ICD are intended as practical tools for mental health-care professionals, beginning with psychiatrists and moving outward from there into the perceptions of wider society. They are not intended as neutral descriptions offered to wider society as starting points for particular cases. Rather, they are intended as neutral descriptions that can be used as explanatory frameworks for all people in all contexts at all times, and in practice that is often how they are perceived.[180] They are constructed specifically as pragmatic responses to particular professional disciplines.

This observation has two consequences. First, it should make those who do not belong to this particular community of reference wary of simply taking up such definitions and applying them as if they were intended as universal explanatory frameworks. Second, the ongoing controversies regarding the construction of these definitions and the ways in which diagnoses and categories shift and change over time should alert us to the subjective and fallible nature of such ways of defining dementia. Cheston and Bender correctly make the point:

> No matter what criteria are developed, the process whereby a diagnosis is reached in inevitably a subjective one carried out by fallible human beings. Moreover, it

is these fallible human beings who have to decide what is and is not an illness. Over time these decisions about illness and symptoms have changed, so that we now recognize sets of behaviors that even 20 years ago would have been disregarded or seen as evidence of moral weakness.[181]

Cheston and Bender highlight the case of ongoing creation of Alzheimer's as indicative of the fallible and political nature of the construction of dementia. For many contemporary people, the term "Alzheimer's disease" has become, at least linguistically, synonymous with dementia. Yet, the complex history of the development of the category of Alzheimer's disease reveals a less-than-straightforward story. Cheston and Bender observe,

> In the 1970s, before the third edition of the DSM, Alzheimer's disease was defined as a pre-senile dementia: an illness which only affected younger people. Later editions of the DSM have defined Alzheimer's disease in a much broader and therefore more inclusive way.... The reasons for this shift are complicated but have much to do with the need to define dementia in a way that will be attractive to potential sources of research money. After all, you can claim to be able to find the cure for a disease in a way that you cannot for old age or senility.[182]

Such a broad interpretation of dementia requires a paradigm shift like that introduced by early Christianity into the Greco-Roman world. The incipient credibility of Christianity in the first century was that it was countercultural—it included Gentiles, Jewish slaves, and male and female Roman citizens—"lepers" that those with dementia have now become in our modern culture. All categories of people were treated as equal persons in Christ. The church, as in days of old, must take such a countercultural stand in the 21st century regarding the unborn child and the senile alike, to treat all as persons, not as cultural artifacts, as wanted and unwanted, useful or useless, legacy or burden. We would argue that even if a demented person requires burdensome care, Christ is able to provide meaning for such care and the courage and capacity to set correct boundaries that protect the care giver and care recipient. But we must be grounded in certain scriptural principles. We are all persons created "in the image of God," whatever our religion or ethnic origins. Yet between the first century and now, little help has been given to the helpless, the insane, and other vulnerable categories of humanity. Admonition to love the least of these helps give biblical purpose and meaning to the hard work of caring for someone who might not recognize or appreciate the care. With earlier diagnoses, the church may need to move into position to prepare those affected by the disease and those who choose to be that loving presence. Though the term caregiver is helpful, it represents a rather modern application of the word that leaves out the word *love*.

As the upheavals of the 14th century show, Western society in the late Middle Ages made virtually no organized provision for the vulnerable members of society other than within a few religious communities.[183] The innovative medical practices from this era have been applied until modern time.[184] Gradually, from the 17th century onward, institutionalized care began to take place. Yet, even in the beginning of the 19th century, medical care for those suffering from mental distress were still being treated as "insane" in conditions worse than prison guard might treat criminals.[185] Most of these mental institutions still remained depersonalizing until the past two or three decades.

Naming dementia as a specific disease makes it more attractive for potential funders. If it is a disease, there might be the possibility of cure. In a socio-culture milieu that tends to fear aging, this can easily be heard and processed in terms of a cure for old age.[186]

This is not to suggest that there is no such thing as Alzheimer's disease, or to in any way downplay it as a valid medical condition. The point is to question the social power of this particular name for dementia. Why is it that one rarely, if ever, finds a high-profile campaign that seek to highlight Lewy bodies, Korsakoff's syndrome, Binswanger's disease, or vascular dementia? Is it coincidental that the disease of Alzheimer's often ends up linguistically representing forms of dementia that are not caused by the specific identifiable disease processes that underpin the diagnosis of Alzheimer's? It may simply be a matter of numbers—more people seem to have Alzheimer's than the other forms of dementia. Even so, we cannot be completely sure about this, because the only way that one can test for Alzheimer's is either postmortem or via medical technology to which most people do not have access. Either that, or it is possible that the more overtly political dimension that Cheston and Bander have noticed is implicitly present within lay and professional discourse.[187] The point is that diagnostic categories are a locus for a complex process of negotiation and a struggle for power and authority that is deeply influenced by such things as cultural expectations, research agendas, and resource allocation. They are considerably less objective and much more flexible than we might or first assume.

The category of dementia is negotiated into existence and sustained by a common agreement and a shared adherence to specific ways of grouping particular forms of human experience. Thus, the shape of dementia inevitably is flexible and permeable, always open to redescription.

Describing Dementia

If we are going to begin the process of redefining dementia, we must first reflect more deeply and critically on the process through which it is currently described and defined. The WHO's ICD-10 defines dementia in this way:

> Dementia is syndrome due to disease of the brain, usually of a chronic or progressive nature, in which there is disturbance of multiple higher cortical functions, including memory, thinking, orientation, comprehension, calculation, learning capability, language, and judgment. Consciousness is not impaired. Impairments of cognitive function are commonly accompanied, occasionally preceded by deterioration in emotional control, social behavior, or motivation. The syndrome occurs in

Alzheimer's disease, in cerebrovascular disease, and in other conditions primarily or secondary affecting the brain.[188]

DSM-IV offers a slightly different description within which chronicity or progression is not required:

A. Impairment in short- and long-term memory.
B. At least one of these:
   1. impairment in abstract thinking
   2. impairment in judgment
   3. other disturbances of higher cortical functioning
   4. personality change
C. That the deficit in A and B significantly interferes with work or social activities.
D. That these deficits should not be caused by delirium.
E. Either there is evidence for the person's history or a physical examination to show that the deficits are produced by a dementia or these problems cannot be accounted for by any other condition.[189]

The story that underpins these definitions appears quite comprehensive, obvious, and clear. Dementia is a brain disease, the product of brain damage brought on by a variety of different causes. This brain damage lead to serious impairment, particularly of the higher cortical functions of brain. This in turn results in cognitive impairment that either causes or is preceded by emotional, behavioral, and motivational problems. Within this narrative of loss and inevitable neutral destruction, the person will lose control of their emotional and social skills, and their ability to interact appropriately will begin to decline, as will their motivation for the tasks of living. The definition does not mention that dementia is a terminal condition or that the person eventually will lose consciousness and die, but the end of the story clearly is not a happy one, even without drawing the terminal nature of dementia to the reader's attention.

From the core descriptions, a series of subcategories of dementia are worked out based on various causal factors. Appendix A outlines some of the main subcategories.[190] The story that underlies these descriptions is precisely the kind of story that guided the doctor in Ignatieff's tale as she tried to describe and explain to the philosopher's son the "true" nature of his mother's condition. This is not surprising, given that the doctor belongs to the group of professionals for whom such descriptions are constructed in the first place. Cheston and Bender suggest that such descriptions reflect what Tom Kitwood has described as the "standard paradigm of dementia":[191]

> The thing that is lost in dementia is defined in terms of the person's intellectual, linguistic, and cognitive functioning. These losses are said to arise directly from neurological impairment, the origins of which are beginning to be identified as having genetic, molecular, and cellular influence. This is, essentially, the representation of dementia in terms of a disease of the brain.[192]

Few would argue that dementia is related to neurological damage. Nonetheless, as will become clear, the power of this is greater than its general accuracy.

Theologians Should Be Wary of Definitions

Given the particular community from which such definitions emerge and feed back into these communities, the tendency toward imperfection should not be surprising. What is surprising are those times when theologians and pastoral caregivers assume that an uncritical acceptance of such descriptions is an appropriate starting point for the development of a specifically Christian theological understanding of dementia. Glen Weaver, a theologian at Calvin College, spends 17 of his 24 pages of his chapter on embodied spirituality in dementia explaining the neurology of dementia, with detailed brain scans.[193] Presumably, he feels that basic knowledge of the condition is necessary for good care and effective theological reflection. Weaver assumes that basic knowledge from the psychiatric community—knowledge that is designed specifically to help that particular community to function according to its internal criteria and goals—is necessarily the best place to begin to reflect theologically on dementia. It is not that such knowledge is necessarily unhelpful; it just might not be the best place for theologians and pastoral caregivers to begin the journey. Beginning with the basic knowledge given to us from the mental health professions, this approach may well feel "natural" and appropriate. It is almost impossible for Western people to think about illness and disease without first thinking about medicine, despite the fact that most healing goes on within the non-professional sectors of the community rather than within professional medicine.[194] Likewise, neurological descriptions of dementia that focus on pathological neurology are turned to first, even though most of the experience of dementia and all of the symptoms of this condition occur in the contexts that emerge, are interpreted within, and lived out quite apart from professional definitions of broken brains. That being so, the desire to begin a theological examination of dementia with an in-depth reflection on the medical story is in some ways understandable.

Nevertheless, one has to ask why a theologian would feel the need to spend significant time laying out an imperfect description of dementia in a non-medical textbook. This seems to be a prime example of starting in the wrong place. What is an appropriate place for the beginning of psychiatry's journey into dementia, however, is not necessarily an appropriate place for theology's journey. In Weaver's article, it is interesting to notice that there are no pictures of people with dementia, and no words are recorded from people experiencing dementia. This absence states quite clearly that communication of this sort is not possible for people with advanced dementia. There is no discussion of potentially central theological contributions to understand dementia, such as grace, dependence, contingency, love, and relationship—aspects that are fundamental to the experience of dementia and fundamental to our understanding of Christian theology. In other words, Weaver assumes throughout his article that theology cannot tell us much about what dementia actually is. That story has been fully narrated and fixed within the standard medical account. The words of neurologists are presented as defining the nature of dementia. Caregivers are given a place to speak on behalf of their loved ones who have dementia, while persons with dementia remain in silence. Theology is brought into reflect on a context that has already been defined by powerful defect-oriented stories that presume they can know what dementia is without knowing persons with dementia.

One can see the tendency to begin with dementia as a medical problem in a good deal of the pastoral literature. On caring for the spiritual needs of people with dementia, Eileen Shamy in her excellent book begins by pointing out that medicine is not her area of expertise. She suggests that she is qualified to provide a detailed study of various conditions that come under the banner of dementia. Nevertheless, she begins the book with what she describes as "key information" about what dementia is:

> Contrary to general belief, dementia is not the name of any disease. Rather, it is a name given to a set of symptoms indicating a need for investigation by a competent doctor trained in this field of medicine.[195]

In this understanding, dementia is a name given to a set of human experiences (symptoms) by doctors who are specially trained in "his field of medicine," the field presumably being some aspect of neurology or psychiatry. It is true that this is an aspect of dementia, but why are the negative aspects of dementia considered to be key aspects, and why, bearing in mind the complex cultural and political contexts that underlie the process of definition, would theologians and pastoral caregivers uncritically accept this description as a given?

We find this medical/imperfect dynamic in what is otherwise an excellent book of essays on dementia edited by Donald McKim, *God Never Forgets: Faith, Hope, and Alzheimer's Disease*.[196] This book is a serious attempt to reflect theologically on dementia and to offer fresh Christian perspectives on this form of human experience—but why does it open with a chapter that focuses on the medical aspects of dementia?

Of course, one could argue that this is necessary in order for people to understand what the condition is and then to respond appropriately to make its points. It is helpful to have the medical perspective.

Patients or Persons

David Keck in his otherwise helpful and theological book on Alzheimer's disease refers to people with dementia as patients.[197] To name persons as patients is to position them in a particular category. Positively, the term "patient" can relate to the ability to bear suffering. It certainly could be argued that this description fits the experience of many people with dementia, particularly in the earlier stages, when the burden of the condition is beginning, but for the most part, the term "patient," at least in common parlance, relates to someone who requires medical care. Why would a theologian desire to identify someone with dementia according to their need for medical care? Most people with dementia are not cared for within healthcare establishments beyond diagnosis, so this seems a rather odd choice of language. The fact that many of us have become trained to associate health and illness with professional medicine is interesting. The fact that we quite often unthinkingly encapsulate such assumptions in the language we use is worrisome. As will become clear, the words we use and the concepts we assume to guide our interpretation of the world and our perceptions of dementia have an impact not just on what we see and do not see, but also on what is actually there. The full impact of this point will become clear later. The thing to keep in mind is that "our words shape our world." Words matter. The language we choose to describe dementia matters immensely.

Redescribing Dementia: Two Interactions

Dementia emerges out of a complicated dialectical interaction between neurological impairment and interpersonal processes.[198] The relationship between neurology and dementia cannot be understood in simple causal terms. Indeed, it may be misleading to say that dementia is a neurological condition if such a statement indicates that the problem lies purely within the confines of an individual's brain. Dementia is closely related to the ways in which society treats particular people and the formation of relationships that exist between these people and society. Dementia may therefore be socially constructed—not only in the sense that it is a diagnostic category arising out of social interaction and discourse by the medical profession—but insofar as it is result of society acting upon individuals in dysfunctional ways.[199] The dysfunction and forgetfulness that mark dementia may in fact reside within the wider community rather than within any particular individual.

Thus, dementia properly should be seen as both neurological and non-neurological. Franzen's belief that his father's actions were nothing more than disease processes that are repeated within millions of other dementia sufferers is true[200] as far as it goes, but it is lacking in explanatory capacity in fundamental ways. In agreement with Kitwood's thinking, dementia is the product of both damaged neurons and the experience of particular forms of relationship and community. The full nature of dementia begins to emerge when we accept that these various elements interact with one another in formative ways.

8

Social and Cultural Stigma—
Negative View of Dementia

"This trail of unraveled brain structure and mounting dysfunction is, in physical terms, only one of inches; yet its silent, implacable wrecking creates entirely new conditions for living life and being with others."
—Arthur Kleinman, *Caregiving: The Soul of Care*[201]

To some extent, our physical illnesses are borne in the context of a socially sick society. City life, intense professional pressure, self-absorbed neighbors, and dysfunctional family life take a toll not only on our spirits but also our bodies. Bereavements, loneliness, labeling, disruption, and many other negative experiences, along with a society already predisposed to alienating senior citizens, add up to an intensely malignant culture for them. Their morale too often dips into a downward spiral to the point that, tragically, some want simply to turn their face to the wall and die. Dementia in its clear stages seems itself to cruelly mock the sufferer; while immediate memory disappears quickly, long term memory often remains intact and so engenders great comparisons and connections between past and present.

Dementia is a significant challenge to the Cartesian assertion, "I think therefore I am!"[202] A senior may not be able any longer to think as lucidly as in the past, nor to remember in ways that satisfy their sense of order and precision. This is why the older years are a time to be loved more than ever before, to dwell in the security of, "I am beloved, therefore I am." The house may now be much more messy, the cooking may sometimes be weird, the day's plan may become less predictable—but so what? These are no longer as important or essential as they previously were thought to be. A "homey home" is what really counts, not a showpiece. It is not dementia that necessarily entails a radical disintegration of the person, but the lack of care for that individual who might no longer experience any love. It is the death of "the person" that is most deadly.

Many unchurched have a personal narrative that explains their later lack of religious support. In the novel, *Still Alice*, when the main character was in the early stage of her disease, the thought of no longer being a Harvard professor terrified her. Almost instinctively, one day, she stumbled into All Saints' Episcopal Church, only a few blocks from her house. She was relieved to find no one there, because she could not explain why she had come. She sat in a pew, looking at the stained glass windows of Jesus, as the shepherd and as the healer performing a miracle. A banner to the right of the altar read, "God is our Refuge and Strength, A Very Present Help in Trouble." She could not be in more trouble than now, so she remained long, waiting for that indefinable "help" to come to her rescue. Her mother had been a secular Jew and she was raised Catholic by her father, so the validity of her childhood faith was never supported by her mother, and she had received no satisfying answers from the church or her father. So now in Alice's trouble, "she felt like a trespasser, undeserving, unfaithful."[203] Similarly, many in our society could find the early stage of dementia a critical opportunity to come to faith, to receive comfort and support where their loss of independence might direct them to a new dimension of hope and comfort. But somehow they come at the wrong time, when the church is empty or with undisclosed barriers of a negative narrative. Or it could be that with senility they cannot bear to confess as did Nicodemus, "How can a man be born? [again] when he is old" (Jn. 3:4).

The Social Construction of Thinking and Humanness

In their research paper titled, "Relationships with Severely Disabled People: The Social Construction of Humanness,"[204] social psychologists Robert Bogdan and Steven Taylor tried to understand the perspectives of non-disabled people who do not stigmatize, stereotype, and reject those with obvious disabilities. Based on their working alongside families with members who have profound intellectual disabilities, Bogdan and Taylor offer some challenging reflections on the ways in which thinking is attributed to family members with disabilities. They begin by noting that "many people with profound intellectual disabilities give few or no obvious signs of experiencing the stimuli presented to them. Most people would say that they lack the ability to think."[205] The non-disabled people in their study, however, believed and, in fact, cited evidence that their disabled partners could and did think, like the philosopher's son in Ignatieff's story, to give the disabled person the benefit of the doubt. Bogdan and Taylor note that "what a person thinks is always subjective and never totally accessible to others."[206] That is the case for all of us—we know what other people think or experience by observing the symbols of speech, writing, gestures, or body language that are meaningful to us. The severely disabled people in Bogdan and Taylor's study were "extremely limited in their abilities to move or make sounds and, hence, to produce symbols. Yet this inability did not prevent their nondisabled partners from attributing thinking to them."[207] According to the authors, the nondisabled people believed that "thinking is different from communicating thought":

> From their perspective, a person can have full thinking
> capacity, be "intelligent" and reflective, but be locked
> in a body that is incapable of or severely limited in its
> capacity for communication. They hold the view that
> their severely disabled partners are more intelligent
> than they appear . . . Attributing thinking to a person
> with or without severe disabilities is a matter of reading
> meaning into the gestures or movements the person

makes. That people with severe disabilities may have a limited repertoire of gestures or movements do not prevent the nondisabled people described in this study from recognizing meaning in gestures and movements they make.[208]

In other words, as insiders who came close to the person on a regular basis, they were noticing things that were invisible to outsiders who popped into the lives of disabled people on a much less intimate level. The tension between the perspectives of the philosopher's son and the doctor highlighted in Ignatieff's story shows this dynamic at work. The distance one has from the person provides the particular hermeneutical framework used to interpret behavior and responses. What one thinks and expects to see is probably what one will end up seeing. Coming close or standing back makes a difference.

Ultimately, what one assumes a person with dementia is thinking will be determined by what one believes is going on within their observed actions and behaviors, and what one *believes* about that will be determined by how one has been taught to understand dementia. In the end, our conclusions ultimately come from the story in which we choose to put our faith. The global and rather vague ascription of "impaired thinking" provides a negative hermeneutic that inevitably will prime a person to see some things and to omit others. Keep in mind, at least within Western cultures, thinking has come to be conceived of as a central dimension of the structure and function of the mind—and, indeed, of what is essential to our humanness. Thus, ascribing impaired thinking to a person with dementia has quite particular connotations: dementia . . . deprived of mind . . . deprived of humanness. The suggestion that a person has impaired thinking might be helpful for a psychologist, but it is much less helpful for a theologian with a critical eye on the implications of uncritically accepting such an apparently obvious statement.

Moving Beyond the Standard Paradigm

The way someone defines things and the expectations that such defining creates will determine what they see and how they respond. This is so with dementia, but it is probably the case with every other thing. The importance of this point has been illustrated well in Franzen's 2001 article in the British newspaper, *The Guardian*, titled, "The Long Slow Slide into the Abyss." This is the story of Jonathan Franzen, born 1959 in Western Spring, Illinois, an America author and essayist of more than ten influential books. He became the first author to appear on the cover of *Time Magazine* since Steven King in 2000. He offers a positive reflection on his experiences with his father, who had Alzheimer's disease. He makes a series of important and quite positive points about the retention of selfhood, the complexities of memory, and the importance of recognizing what remains available when people go through dementia. Toward the end of the article, his tone begins to change as he starts to reflect differently on his father's experience. He developed his more positive perspective on dementia since he was young. As he grew older and wiser, thing looks different:

> Fretting about what a self-righteous 30-year-old I was, I can see my reluctance to apply to my father the term of Alzheimer's to protecting the specific of Earl Franzen from the generality of a nameable condition. Conditions have symptoms; symptom point to an organic basis of everything we are. They point to brain as meat. I seem instead to maintain a blind spot across which I interpolate stories that emphasize the soul-like aspects of self. Seeing my afflicted father as a set of organic symptoms would invite me to understand the healthy Earl Franzen in symptomatic terms as well—to reduce our beloved personalities to finite sets of neurological coordinates. Who wants a story of life like that?[209]

The young Franzen was reluctant to take the suggestion that the organic basis of all human existence determines what human beings are. He recognized that ascribing the label "Alzheimer's" to his father's behavior would diminish his specificity and draw all that he was into the totalizing power of the diagnosis. Instead, he focused on those aspect of his father's experience that he considered to be "soul-like," by which he presumably meant, among other things, not wholly explicable by or reducible to neurological changes. With the passage of time, however, he learned to see things differently:

> For now, I feel uneasy when I gather facts about Alzheimer's. Reading David Shenk's new book, *The Forgetting: Alzheimer's: Portrait of an Epidemic*, I am reminded that when my father got lost in his own neighborhood, or forgot to flush the toilet, he was exhibiting symptoms identical to those of millions of other affected people. . . . I am sorry to see the personal significance drain from certain mistakes of my father's, like his confusion of my mother with her mother, which struck me at the time as singular and orphic, and from which I gleaned all manner of important new insight into my parent's marriage. My sense of private selfhood turns out to have been illusory.[210]

Finally persuaded by the explanatory lure of the medical story, Franzen saw things differently. As a consequence, his perceptions of the thoughts and actions of his father shifted—gone were the apparently idealistic hopes that his father's actions might be meaningful and undetermined by failing neurology. He had come to realize that his father's behavior was nothing more than the symptoms that are experienced by countless other people with Alzheimer's disease. His father's private actions had become public "symptoms" of a most feared disease. The story of his experience with his father shifted in quite profound ways.[211]

Franzen's story is not much different than many others. He changed his mind because he was persuaded by a story that was more powerful than his initial story of hope and "soulishness." He changed his mind back again, because there was good reason for it—if his father's condition were described and understood properly, there was a reason for hope. Franzen's reflections on father's experience were both correct and incorrect— dementia is *not* neurological; dementia is not only or, perhaps, not even *primarily* neurological. Such paradoxical statements seem somewhat counter-intuitive. How can the answer be both yes and no? Dementia is neurological, but it is much more than that. There are similarities among the experiences of people with dementia, but there are no "typical dementia patients." Even those similarities that do exist may not always relate to similar changes within individual brains. Something else is going on, such that the definition of dementia needs to be expanded; there is a need of counter-story.

To Die or not to Die

Moving on from lay perceptions of personhood into the world of academic philosophy, people see that the seemingly instinctual response, "Shoot me if I get like that," finds more poignant yet blunt expression. In a 2008 interview with the Presbyterian Church of Scotland's magazine *Life and Work*, Baroness Mary Warnock raised sharply the issue of personhood in people with dementia. Reflecting on why she had left instructions with her solicitor and doctor expressing a desire not to be resuscitated if/when she were dying, she moves on to talk about dementia with the interviewer:

> "The real fear, I think shared with nearly everyone, is that I become demented. I've left instructions that if I contract pneumonia or something that I'm not to be given antibiotics, but there's not much else I can do.... *If you're demented, you're wasting people's lives*—your family's lives—and you're wasting the resources of the National Health Service."

> I [the interviewer] point out to her that the argument for euthanasia usually revolves around pain, and that people with dementia are not normally subject to great pain.

"I don't think that's the full argument," she says, shaking her head. "I'm absolutely fully in agreement that if pain is insufferable then someone should be given help to die, but I feel there's a wider argument that if somebody absolutely, desperately wants to die because they're a burden to their family or the state, then I think they too should be allowed to die.[212]

Actually, Warnock makes a case for advanced directives wherein a person could appoint an advocate to ensure that their life was ended under certain circumstances:

I think that's the way the future will go. Putting it rather brutally, you'd be licensing people to put others down. Actually, I think why not, because the real person has gone already and all that's left is just the body of a person, and nobody wants to be remembered in this condition.[213]

The negative and malicious ways in which people with dementia are positioned within Warnock's comments are far from subtle. According to her, people with dementia are a burden to their families, the National Health Service, and the state. They're wasting other people's lives and should have the decency to take their own lives. In a somewhat grotesque parody of Jesus' statement, "There is no greater love than to lay down your life for a friend," Warnock suggests that suicide is morally appropriate if one feels that it is the best thing for other people. One can only imagine how a person recently diagnosed with dementia might feel upon reading her words.

Warnock's comments provoked outrage and concern among many, with Alzheimer Scotland asking: "Why dementia, distinct from other illnesses, should be considered a 'burden' to the NHS and to society?"[214] Why indeed? The answer is quite simple, especially since cancer, pneumonia, and appendicitis are not perceived as affecting one's personhood. The key to Warnock's position lies in her final sentence:

the real person has gone, and the body is all that remains. Philipa Malpas sums this position well:

> What Warnock actually seems to be suggesting is that being a person is what really matters in the context of those elderly afflicted by dementia. It is not that I have a duty to die because I have dementia and am a burden to others; rather, it is because I am no longer a person. I am just a body.[215]

According to this viewpoint, the individual diagnosed with dementia has begun making a transition from being a person to being a non-person. As a non-person, she has no right to the kinds of moral respect and protection to which she might otherwise be entitled. That being so, to kill her is considered appropriate; if she kills herself, it is convenient.

Redefining Dementia: Two Important Views

Two primary views describe dementia, the two creators of which have been deeply influential in providing the basis for this book's counter-story—they are psychologists Tom Kitwood from U.K. and Steven Sabat from U.S. Both in different but deeply connected ways have challenged the standard story of dementia and offered important alternative ways of looking at, describing, and defining dementia. For both, dementia is as much *relational* and *social* as it is neurological. The two are inseparable for a proper understanding of dementia, since one needs to look beyond dementia, and beyond neurology, toward the complex network of relationship that surround the person who is the recipient of the diagnosis.

A key point is that relationships may be important for more reasons than simply because it is not good that people with dementia should be alone (it is not). Rather, the assertion is that relationships may be both causative and formative within the development of the syndrome of experiences and neurological damage that forms dementia. In other words, relationships are part of what dementia actually is, not just an aspect of how we should offer care to people once the nature of the condition has been defined. Both Kitwood and Sabat want to expand the definition of what dementia is to include the significance of such things as love, relationships, and care. This, for the author, is a much stronger and more appropriate place for theology and pastoral care to begin the journey into dementia. Let us begin by thinking through the implications of Kitwood's suggestion that dementia has to do with relational disorder and his attempts to develop what he describes as a "neurology of personhood,"[216] that is, a model of what he describes as a personhood, which recognizes and seeks to bring to the fore the intimate connection between neurology and social experience.

Connection between Dementia and Malicious Social Psychology

Kitwood's point in re-narrating the causal factors that lie behind the development of dementia is twofold (see also Appendix D). First, he wants to loosen the hold that the standard paradigm has on our understanding of dementia and create a space for a different approach that takes care and relationship as seriously as neurological decline, deficit, and damage. He wants to initiate a new story that will present a new worldview. Second, he wants people to realize that they may be implicit in the creation of the symptoms of dementia. No longer can we avoid responsibility for dementia by blaming it all on neurology. If Kitwood is correct, then society may well have a profound responsibility for causing the symptoms of Dementia rather than simply responding to them. The symptoms of Franzen's father might not only have been more than a particular manifestation of a generalized syndrome; they may also have been the product and manifestation of the society within which he lived, breathed, and experienced dementia.

In making the claim that relationships are in fact central to what dementia is, Kitwood wishes to make us aware of the ways in which people relate to those who have dementia and implications that such relating has for the development of the condition physically, psychologically, and socially. In particular, Kitwood wants his readers to notice the profoundly negative ways in which relationships with people who have dementia often work themselves out. The term "dementia" does not just describe a set of symptoms. It also describes a quite particular way of being in the world that has cultural significance. To become deeply forgetful amid elevating intellect and reason over other aspects of being human has quite specific meaning, and that meaning is deeply negative. Stephen Post puts it this way:

> We live in a culture that is the child of rationalism and capitalism, so clarity of mind and economic productivity determine the value of human life. The dictum "I think, therefore I am" is not easily replaced with "I will, feel, and relate while disconnected by forgetfulness from my former self, but I am." Neither cogito (I think) nor ergo (therefore), but sum (I exist). Human beings are much more than sharp minds, powerful remembrances, and economic successes.[217]

Post identifies the key problem for people with dementia living within such a cultural milieu as the general tendency toward *hypercognition*.[218] This idea relates to the tendency within Western cultures to isolate intellect, reason, and rationality and identify these aspects of human beings as having particular moral and social significance.[219] In this view, a life that is truly valuable and worth living is fundamentally defined by the ability to function effectively on the level of intellect and reason. Such hypercognitive cultures inevitably will construct dementia in particularly negative terms. This construction necessarily will impact how people respond to those who receive the name "dementia." Thus, there is an explicit and implicit negative cultural bias toward diseases that involve deterioration in intellect, rationality, autonomy, and freedom, which are those facets of human beings that Western cultures have chosen to value over and above others. It is Kitwood's intention to sensitize us to the clinical and relational implications of such negative psychological and sociological processes.

Kitwood suggests that this cultural bias means that many who are programmed to think of dementia negatively, which inevitably means that their relationships with people who bear the diagnosis have a tendency toward negativity. He offers a story:

> Concerning the failure of the photographic exercise from the standpoint of agency who promotes awareness about Alzheimer's disease of a *day center* for publicity purpose. The agency rejected the photographs on the ground that the clients did not show the disturbed and agonized characteristics that people with dementia "ought" to show, and which would be expected to arouse public concern was a measure of the success of the day care from the standpoint of clients. Here the clients with dementia were continuing to live in the world of persons, and not being downgraded into the carriers of an organic brain disease. Devalued the person and make a unique and sensitive human being into an instance of some category devised for convenience or control.[220]

The tension between the hypercognitive cultural story with its expectations and demands for loss and devastation to be the prevailing script and counter-story of love and possibilities could not be more striking. Kitwood names such negative relational processes forms *malignant social psychology* or MSP (I will use malicious instead). The term refers to social environments in which the forms of interpersonal interactions and communications that occur diminish the personhood of those people experiencing that malignant environment.[221]

An example of MSP would be not thinking twice about talking about people as if they were not there: "He won't remember!"; "She can't understand"; "He isn't really the person he used to be"; and so on. Of course, they do not know the truth of any these statements; they are simply assumptions made based on the content and meaning that have been ascribed to the name "dementia" and presumptions that have been made about the connection between dementia and "loss of mind and self."

Similarly, some might find themselves making comparisons between the individual with dementia and a child: "She's just like a child. It's like caring for a one-year-old." But of course she is not "just like a child." Even if her behavior does seem analogically childlike, she is an adult with a history and a story that make her who she is. She is not growing into and learning about the world as a child does. Even if her brain can no longer hold onto memories, her body remains formed and available in a world that has bodily familiarity, even if that familiarity can no longer be named. At that point, someone will be taking her to a care home where she will spend the rest of her life with strangers. All of these things are examples of not giving people the benefit of doubt. As will become clear, there is in fact plenty of room for doubt.

Malicious interactions need not be perpetrated out of malice. Oftentimes, they occur because of thoughtlessness, lack of insight, or lack of awareness about the negative effects of particular attitudes, actions, behaviors, and relationships. Frequently, they are the product of underlying cultural assumptions about worth and value. When we are taught to see people with dementia in particular ways, we assume that we should respond to demented accordingly. Because we tend to look *through* rather than *at* things we are taught about dementia, we often have no way of knowing how destructive some of our everyday assumptions and attitudes actually are. All of these things have the cumulative effect of depersonalizing individuals with dementia and placing them in situations where relationships subtly and sometimes rapidly move from "I-Thou" to "I-it"; from the personal to the objectified impersonal. The implication here is that it is malformed relationships rather than pure neurology that lie behind many of the symptoms and experience of dementia. If that is so, it may be that a changed relational context might bring about changed behavior and reduction in symptoms If this is so, then we should be concentrating as much on care as on neurology. Relationships and care need to become aspects of how we describe, define, and seek to understand dementia.

Kitwood summarizes his overall position and revised definition of dementia in the form of an equation: D (Dementia) = NI (Neurological Impairment) + PH (Physical Health) + B (Biography) + MSP (Malicious

Social Psychology). They are all related with each other and impacted to each other. In this equation, the particular neurological configurations that have occurred function in various ways in developing the brain's structure and architecture, thus accounting for variation in resilience to the process of dementia. In order to understand the experience of dementia, we first need to understand the person's story.[222] The experience of dementia is in turn deeply impacted by the person's experience of MSP. It is as these various elements interact with each another that the full nature of dementia begins to emerge. Experience and biography matter for the ways in which we conceptualize, understand, and respond to dementia (for further discussion, see Appendix D)

"Excess Disability" and Malicious Social Positioning

Steven Sabat takes up, develops, and in important ways offers further verification of Kitwood's thinking in the idea of *excess disability*:

> there has been considerable reason to have at least some doubt that the myriad symptoms observed in AD sufferers are due to brain pathology alone. More than 25 years ago Brody terms *excess disability* to describe what he calls the "the discrepancy that exists when a person's functional incapacity is greater than that warranted by the actual impairment."[223]

> If that is the case, there would seem to be only one possible realm in which that disability is rooted, and that would be the social world in which the person with AD dwells.[224]

Excess disability relates to manifestations of incapacity that do not relate directly to any physical damage that might have occurred to an individual. Schizophrenia from social isolation and exclusion, for example, emerges not only from the condition itself but from people's reaction to the label.[225] Schizophrenia is certainly debilitating, but much of the disability is excessive, that is epiphenomenal to the syndrome itself. The same is true of dementia—excess disability relates to malicious social psychology in that one leads into the other.

For Sabat, the problem is that people cannot see such excessive disability with the standard approach, which is not designed to recognize it. Therefore, excess disability becomes invisibly grafted into the standard paradigm and seemingly "disappears." Sabat notes,

> the tragic irony here: however objective and useful the standard approach may be in certain venues, it is relatively insensitive contexts of the social world in which of us, including the afflicted, live our lives. Yet on the basis of results of research using the standard paradigm, they have planted a mosaic, created a narrative, about the afflicted person's ability in the very social world which is not studied through that research. In other words, on the basis of the standard approach, incorrect negative assumptions can be made by those who interact with AD sufferers in the everyday social world.[226]

The place where Sabat notices such negative assumptions is in the language that is used about and around people with dementia. His central concept, which captures the dynamics of this process is the idea of "malicious social positioning," which draws from Kitwood's idea of malicious social psychology, adding to it the theory of social positioning. The effects of dementia derive from a neurological changed brain of the person thus

> diagnosed and can be exacerbated or ameliorated to some degree by the way the person is positioned by others in the everyday social world. By analyzing the nature of their social interactions with others, we can readily come to appreciate how the ways in which the person with dementia is treated by others can have profoundly positive or profoundly negative effect on: 1)

the subjective experience of the person with dementia;
2) the degree to which the person can display remaining
interactive cognitive abilities; 3) the ability of the person
to meet the demands of everyday life, and 4) the quality
of the person's social life and the meaning found in each
day.[227]

In the thinking of psychologist Rom Harré and his revision
of traditional role theory, human role relationships are expressed
through language. He criticizes standard notions of roles as being
overly static, disembodied, and paying little attention to specifics of
what Sabat calls positioning theory.[228] Thus, Harré provides a way
to read and understand the dynamics of contexts. Roles describe
typical positions but fail to identify the particular experience of
someone who is ascribed such a role. Positioning theory thus offers a
more dynamic perspective than role theory, focusing on the special
position of an individual within an encounter. How a person's position
within a relationship is oriented will determine how they respond
to others and also will reveal what others think of the person, even
if such things are unspoken. A person's position in any encounter is
communicated through language. Malicious social positioning occurs
when a person is positioned in such a way within a social encounter
that their personhood is threatened.[229]

Imagine a wife introducing her husband to others as a person with
dementia. One can see how the husband is positioned in a particular way,
given all of the roles that he has in his life. The wife chooses linguistically
to position him as a dementia sufferer, which means that his normal role
as a husband is significantly weakened and negatively transformed. He
also lost his multifaceted role as a functional husband and has acquired a
primary identity as someone who has dementia. For Sabat, this sense of
depersonalizing position is malicious:

> Position help to define, strengthen, or weaken a person's
> moral and personal attributes and help to create story-
> lines about persons. Through the process of positioning,

people explain their own behavior that emphasize the individual's negative attributes is to position that person in a potentially malignant way.[230]

Lisa Snyder's ethnographic work in a home for people with dementia.[231] Sabat offers a powerful example of this process of malignant positioning:

> Betty, a retired social worker and former faculty member at San Diego State University talked about health care professionals' un-receptiveness to the significance of illness for people whom she encounters during the process of her being diagnosed. They know the diagnosis, but they don't take time to know what that truly means for that person. Especially when they deal Alzheimer's. We have to be really willing to be present with the person who has Alzheimer's disease; their casualness is painful to see. . . . But there are some people who don't want to learn, it is the looking down on and being demeaning of people with Alzheimer's that is hard to watch.[232]

To position Betty as a "dementia patient" is to take away her many primary roles and to replace them with a psychiatric category. The category makes sense because it does its work within the healthcare system, but it makes little sense when Betty is home, or as she tries to make sense of her world within a care home or sheltered accommodation. When we become our illness, our very humanness is threatened. Snyder commended poignantly, "A person with Alzheimer's disease is many more things than just their diagnosis, each person is a whole human being."[233] Sabat offers this strong denunciation of malignant positioning of people like Betty:

> Once persons are positioned socially as nothing more than instantiations of diagnostic category, their essential humanity, including their intellectual and emotional characteristics, needs, and their social personae beyond

that of "demented, burdensome patient" become more
and more obscured and can ultimately become erased.[234]

In introducing the idea of malicious positioning, Sabat draw our attention to the fact that the language people use reflects the stories they are utilizing to make sense of the person with dementia. In doing so, Sabat expands on Kitwood's suggestion of a general malicious social psychology and focuses on the particular ways in which this positioning is manifested—in subliminal attitudes expressed through language that maliciously positions people in ways that threaten their very humanness (for further discussion, see Appendix D).

9

Hospitality among Strangers: Christian Community as a Place of Belonging

"The strangers who dwell among you shall be to you as one born among you, and you shall love him as yourself; for you were strangers in the land of Egypt: I am the Lord your God." (Leviticus 19:34, NKJV)

"So now you Gentiles are no longer strangers and foreigners. You are citizens along with all of God's holy people. You are members of God's family." (Ephesians 2:19)

"Who am I or who I am?" Ultimately, the answer to the question lies in the hands of God. Dementia no longer is to be feared not in the way it was feared before. For those who experience dementia later in life, much of who they thought they were and much of what others think they are will slip away as the neurological damage shifts and changes the expressions of themselves. They can and probably will be anxious, angry, and disappointed, but they do not have to be afraid as long as they are certain that God will remember them, and that memory has active power for the present and future. They need not be afraid as long as they are certain that those whom they love—family, friends, and community—and the people of God's memory in the church, will continue to love and remember them. As long as they know that they can trust in God and in those who love them to remember them well, they will be safe.

But there is still one nagging question that needs to be explored. It is all well and good for people to expect others to remember and love them. But what they are actually asking others to do is to keep loving them even when who they are becomes difficult. To ask people to continue to love them for who they are in such condition is a pretty big request. To ask others to love the one who is sick is always difficult. But to ask others to love and care for them when they become so different from the one who originally was so loved, may seem impossible. What might it mean to love this *stranger* who was so loved before?

Becoming Stranger

What is it about dementia that turns people into strangers? People with dementia can quickly discover that part of their changing identity relates to their becoming strangers both to themselves and to others. Thomas DeBaggio, in his autobiography, *Losing My Mind: An intimate Look at Life with Alzheimer's*, lays out a painful, moving, and often angry account of what it is like to journey into dementia:

> Alzheimer's sends you back to an elemental world before time, a world devoid of possibility and secrets. It is a world of insecurity where the certainty of words and memory of events is unstable. It is a world of abject insecurity and tears and frustration. I sense reality slipping away, and words become slipping sand. My life is turning into a dun-colored kaleidoscope. I think it will be only a matter of months before my life becomes a nightmare and the world become a freshly unknowable place where even the simplest things are difficult because they are unrecognizable.[235]

As DeBaggio loses his sense of who he is and what the world is like, he finds himself a stranger to both himself and the world. Dementia is a series of small deaths that strip the peace from his previously hopeful life, casting him adrift in a world that is rapidly vanishing:

> There is a wide emotional difference between knowing you will die one day in the future and living with knowledge you have a disease that slowly squeezes the life from you in hundreds of unexpected ways, and you have to watch it happen while those who love you stand by unable to help you.[236]

DeBaggio is lonely and helpless. Those around him are lonely and helpless—onlookers and witnesses to the demise of the one they knew and the emergence of a stranger. Every time he goes to sleep, he realizes, "this may be my last chance to dream."[237] His fear is not that he will die; his fear is that he no longer will remember what it is like to live.

Forgetting Who We Are and Whose We Are

One of the most profound and moving Christian testimonies about what it is like to experience dementia is found in Robert Davis's autobiography, *My Journey into Alzheimer Disease*. Pastor of a mega church in Miami, Florida, a powerful preacher and dynamic minister, it gradually became obvious to Davis that things were not right. He was forgetting, becoming confused. He could not cope with the responsibilities on which he once thrived. When he was diagnosed with Alzheimer's disease, it shook the very foundation of his faith. His book offers insight into what it means to be moving into the advanced stages of Alzheimer's as well as insight into what it means to try to hold onto faith and love as all of one's old certainties slowly slip away.

Davis began his journey holding onto Jesus and feeling assured that God was in control. But soon things became increasingly difficult as the spiritual resources that carried him on his journey began to fail:

> My spiritual life was still miserable. I could not read the
> Bible. I could not pray as I wanted because my emotions
> were dead and cut off. . . . My mind also raced about,
> grasping for the comfort of the Savior whom I knew and
> loved and for the emotional peace that he could give me,
> but finding nothing. I concluded that the only reason for
> such darkness must be spiritual. Unnamed guilt filled
> me. Yet the only guilt I could put a name to was failure
> to read my Bible. But I could not read, and would God
> condemn me for that? I could only lie there and cry, "Oh
> God, why? Why?"[238]

Davis was becoming a stranger. The things that held him steady
in the world—his faith, his love for Jesus, and his sense of identity as
a Christian—were all beginning to slip away. The resources that he
depended on to hold onto his faith were not functioning properly because
of his neurological decline. He was losing himself, and his greater fear was
that he was losing God, too. The resonance between Davis's lament and
the words of Psalm 88 is obvious:

> I call to you, O Lord, every day;
> I spread out my hands to you.
> ....
> Why, O Lord, do you reject me
> And hide your face from me? (vv. 9–14)

The process of becoming a stranger, to yourself, to others, and to
God, is a long and painful one.

Watching Helplessly

DeBaggio's comment on the helplessness of the onlooker raises important
issues. Davis's autobiography is frequently quoted within the pastoral
literature on dementia, and rightly so. It is a powerful story about the
experience of Alzheimer's and the role of faith, Spirit, and hope. But

attention has been paid to Davis's wife, Betty, who wrote the book with her husband and, presumably, gradually took on a more prominent role as his condition progressed. Her voice is formally silent until the epilogue. At that point she explodes onto the scene as herself:

> Some time I feel like God's special pet—held in that special place of all those who are called to share "the fellowship of his suffering." Sometimes I feel like Jesus in the Garden, "Please, if it be your will, let this cup pass— let me wake up to learn all this is just a bad dream and all is as before . . . will this be the night from which reason will never again awaken? Will morning find that new person in my bed—the man who will not know who I am or why I am in his bed?[239]

Dementia indeed evokes lament.[240]

Why, My God?

Aileen Barclay, an essayist[241] whose husband has Alzheimer's disease, offers some insights into the role that lament might play in coming to terms with the losses of dementia. The following is her extended meditation on Psalm 88, reflecting on her experience with her husband:

> In despair, confusion, and the grief of living with my husband, who once was a capable, intelligent, and gracious man, I remember the person whom I married and with whom I share my life. I withdraw from my lively church, just unable to face people who keep telling me what a wonderful person my husband is. Nonetheless, physical withdrawal from church does not mean that God withdraws, even though it may often feel as if he has. "Your wrath lies heavily upon me" wails the psalmist, conjuring up images of those six silent hours as Jesus hung on the cross when all seemed lost, broken, fractured.

You have taken from me my closest friends
And have made me repulsive to them
I am confined and cannot escape. (v. 8)

From the cross, Jesus' loneliness is a stark reminder to us. We, too, have become repulsive to our friends and cut off from the community, suffering from the terrors of night. Darkness has indeed become our closest friend. Lacking the cognitive abilities to participate in social life or overstepping the unwritten rules of social conventions, one-time friends no longer seek our company. Invitations to dinner at our home, once eagerly accepted, are "postponed" with lame excuses. Aileen learns that she no longer is part of a couple—that honored institution of the church that opens doors of friendship and fellowship. She learns that she is not single, either, and thus cannot find solace among the women who complain that the church only has time for those who are married.

My eyes are dim with grief.
I call to you, O, Lord, every day;
I spread out my hands to you. (v. 9)

Her husband's dementia has turned Aileen from a wife and a friend into a stranger. Friends no longer seem to recognize her. She is married but not married; in the community of the church but not fully of that community; single yet not a single. Experiencing social strangeness and caring for someone with dementia also revealed to Aileen her own inner strangeness, which emerged as she gradually became aware that the person she thought she was, was not the person she actually was or had become. She quotes from Psalm 88:

From my youth I have been afflicted and close to death,
I have suffered your terrors and am in despair.
...
You have taken my companion and loved ones from me;
The darkness is my closest friend. (15:1)

In the darkness of the night, she remembers who she truly is, the mistakes she has made, the deliberate actions and justifications to get her own way, to remain in control. She remembers the lasting consequences of her thoughts, intentions, and actions, suffering the terrors, despairing that for the all years she had claimed to be part of God's eternal kingdom, but as a caregiver she feels she is failing to live up to the love, joy, and peace that first attracted her to Jesus. She senses God's wrath weighing heavily upon her, flooding her sleeping and waking hours, engulfing her under a mighty wave of reproach. Her self-centeredness, her complaints, her continued anger with her increasingly frail husband all lead to alienation from others, unable to cope with her endless outpouring of grievances. Their thoughtless remarks remind her of how she is being reconstructed.

> If he stays with you, you'll kill him,
> You only speak about your own needs!
> This is your burden—you have to get on with it.
> I am not interested in your needs—your husband is my client.
> We have all got different personalities—you don't have the right one to care for a person with Alzheimer's.

Aileen knew her husband had the disease years before his diagnosis. The deterioration had been a slow but relentless destruction of his capacities as a competent adult. He had become a frightened child, petulant and manipulative, dependent upon her for what little order can be created around his disappearing capacities. "It is like carrying around on my back a weight that is too heavy for the scale. The pendulum has swung so far that the plate, like a broken swing, has hit the ground."[242]

Aileen's reflections on the Psalm of lament ended in her own lament as she gradually began to see that both she and her husband had become strangers in the eyes of others and increasingly strangers in their own eyes. Dementia brings suffering with it, and that suffering creates strangers in many senses of the word.

Beyond Suffering

Dementia brings suffering both to the person diagnosed with the disease and to those who seek to offer care and support, which is a particular kind of suffering. Arthur Kleinman, a social anthropologist who cares for his Alzheimer-stricken wife, comments, "We have marked by a special kind of pain."[243] Dementia is a form of *affliction*. Simone Weil, in her book *Waiting on God*, offers an understanding of affliction:

> In the realm of suffering, affliction is something apart, specific, irreducible. It is quite a different thing from simple suffering. It takes possession of the soul and marks it through and through with its own particular mark, the mark of slavery.[244]

Affliction involves physical pain of particular kind, such as toothache, painful but it passes away. The pain of affliction is enduring, drawn out, and deeply impacts the whole person:

> There is not real affliction unless the event which has seized and uprooted a life attacks it, directly or indirectly, in all parts, social, psychological, and physical. The social factor is essential. There is no really affliction where there is not social degradation or the fear of it in some form or another.[245]

This is clearly what De Baggio experienced:

> With any untreatable, disabling malady, the victims become sensitized to every movement of their body, every breath, searching for change and studying the course of the illness until it threatens to destroy friendships and the love of those around them.[246]

Dementia may not be marked by physical pain, but it is a deeply painful experience in all of the dimensions Weil highlights. Affliction can produce self-hatred, self-contempt, and feelings of guilt.[247] Aileen's sensing of those aspects of herself that were less than perfect emerged from and reflected her experience of affliction, which also impacted her sense of God's presence:

> Affliction makes God appear to be absent for a time, more absent than a dead man, more absent than light in the utter darkness of a cell. A kind of horror submerges the whole soul. During the absence there is nothing to love. What is terrible is that if, in this darkness where there is nothing to love, the soul ceases to love, God's absence becomes final.[248]

This was clearly Davis's experience and the psalmist's experience as well. While some forms of affliction can be eased by a change in circumstances, the terrifying thing about the affliction that accompanies dementia is that there is no real possibility of it moving on. The psalmist's cry—"You have taken my companions and loved ones from me, the darkness is my closest friend"—has an eternal quality that is deeply disturbing. Unlike other Psalms of lament, Psalm 88 offers no hopeful return to God—only darkness.

The problem with affliction is that it is isolating and alienating. Only those who are or who have been afflicted can understand what it means. It is not possible to project one's self directly into the situation of the afflicted. One can only think through what it might mean for them. As Eric Springsted puts it,

> Affliction, however, is much more difficult to imagine because in affliction we actually lose ourselves. This is why we also do not usually even notice the afflicted; what we think we see is a person who is in need of help, or who needs to pull himself up by his bootstraps. But in fact, there is no person left there to help.[249]

Springsted does not mean that the person literally ceases to exist. The point he wants to make is that the affliction overwhelms people so they lose sight of who they are; psychologically they struggle to exist. For people with dementia, this relates to their feeling that somehow their true selves are fading away—even though, as has been shown, this is not at all the case. For caregivers, it has to do with the way in which their caring role subsumes every other role and every possibility for their lives. The affliction become all that they are, and they become slaves to their conditions. All parties involved—caregivers and care recipients—become strangers to themselves and to others, lost within their afflictions without the resources to rescue themselves:

> You have put me in the lowest pit,
> In the darkest depths.
> Your wrath lies heavily upon me;
> You have overwhelmed me with all your wave.
> You have taken from me my closet friends
> And have made me repulsive to them.
> I am confined and cannot escape;
> My eyes are dim with grief. (Ps. 88:6–9)

The affliction of dementia makes strangers of ourselves and the ones we love.

The Passion—the Pain and Affliction—of Christ

The affliction that is experienced by those who are marked by dementia is echoed in the divine affliction revealed paradigmatically in the passion of Christ. Weil points to Jesus' passion as the place where divine affliction is most poignantly revealed. Clearly, Jesus was afflicted in all the senses that have been discussed, and yet he continued to love. Perhaps Jesus' greatest sense of affliction came when he was abandoned, or at least experienced the feeling of being abandoned. Yet even in the void, Jesus kept on loving. It is here we begin to see some possibilities for hope. Springsted makes an interesting observation:

> Even though Jesus could neither see nor understand anything that corresponded to the good he had set out to accomplish, he still continued to love in the void that was left and refused to deny that love. Jesu did not mistakenly identify that good with any earthly good, nor try to find any compensation for his sufferings, as we often try to do to remedy our sufferings. He simply remained as far removed from the Father as anyone could be and continue to love. Even though God was utterly absent, Jesus still loved and remained faithful, although he had no hope.[250]

In the passion and affliction of Jesus, we can see pain, loss, abandonment, and deep lament, which in a real sense mirrors the experience of dementia for caregivers and care recipients: "My God, my God, why have you forsaken me?"[251] is a mode of speech that comes naturally to afflicted people. And yet in and through the pain and affliction of Jesus, we encounter "redemption." Even in the apparent absence of God, Weil observes, Jesus' love is in no way diminished. The passion of Christ opens up the possibility that even though what we see does not at all correspond with what we think we should be seeing, and what we truly desire to be seeing, love remains possible. And redemption can be achieved. This could be expressed as a sharp caution: "Don't believe that which seems to be apparent!" Even as our prayers seem to scream into a silent abyss, the resurrection for which the passion was a necessity puts new meaning into Jesus' words: "You parents, if your children ask for a loaf of bread, do you give them a stone instead?" (Matt. 7:9). Even when our prayers seem not to be answered, the assurance that Jesus continues to love us provides a basis for faithful hopefulness and gives a particular shape to our sufferings. How can affliction be overcome? Through love. From whence does such love come? From Jesus.

Like other crucial aspect of the experience of dementia, however—memory, mind, identity—such faith in the face of affliction cannot be achieved alone. Overcoming the alienation, isolation, and enforced strangerhood that accompanies the experience of dementia cannot be done without friends and without community who have learned to recognize the value of strangers, and who can acknowledge the reality of the experience of affliction and, in so doing, bring healing and new hope. Affliction can destroy love and force us to look at people in the wrong way. Affliction is a breeding ground for malicious social psychology and negative positioning by ourselves and others. What is required is a community that can offer emphatic hospitality to strangers, a community that truly sees the experiences of dementia for what they are, a community that has the time and resources to move people from affliction to hope: from strangeness to belonging.

Fear of Strangers

Dementia creates strangers; love overcomes strangeness. Love, then, is central to the creation of the types of relationships that Kitwood and Sabat have shown are central for understanding dementia and providing person-centered dementia care. Malicious social psychology and native positioning tend to typify the way in which we react to strangers. We fear strangers, and we seek way to distance ourselves from them. To be a stranger is to be a threat to the cohesion and safety of a group or community. To be an afflicted stranger is to be someone whom others do not and indeed cannot understand. We also do not understand those who choose to be with the afflicted, or those who have no choice other than to be with them. This was one of Jesus' problems. Because he spent time with strangers—those sinful persons—their stigma and alienation became his. "The Son of Man came eating and drinking, and you say. Here is a glutton and a drunkard, a friend of tax collectors and 'sinners.'" It sometimes seems that strangers rub off on those who hang around with them.

Turning people into strangers is one way of creating distance and safety. A stranger threatens the settled agreement within a community about what is good, bad, normal, and abnormal. It is much easier to push strangers to the margins and carry on as before than it is to answer the challenge that they brings with them. It is easier to offer charity to people with dementia than it is to offer welcome. Charity can mean giving alms to strangers—holding them at arm's length but convincing ourselves that we are acting compassionately. Welcome requires embrace and rarely do we willingly embrace strangers. Above all else, the stranger threatens our peacefulness, our sense of *shalom*. People with dementia threaten hypercognitive perception of *shalom* in deep ways. If *shalom* has to do with righteous, holiness, and right relationship with God,[252] and if the orthodox way of knowing God is assumed primarily to be cognitive and intellectual, then those who come proclaiming that the standard ways of relating to God might not apply to them inevitably will create a dissonance that at best is disorienting and at worst is offensive. It is easier to position people with dementia as strangers whose customs, worldviews, and experiences are alien to us; it might be easier for us to acknowledge their value in their differences than to face the challenge of what it might mean to love God when we no longer know God is. Clearly, people with dementia bring strangeness in a myriad of ways and sit neatly within the role of stranger both culturally and spiritually.

Hospitality to Strangers

Recognizing the ways in which those involved with dementia become strangers is the first step toward developing a way of looking at their strangeness in terms of healing possibilities. The idea of offering hospitality to the stranger is a key theme that runs throughout both Old and New Testaments.[253] The Hebrew Bible provides three terms for the stranger: *ger, nochri, and zar.* In brief, they must be treated the way we have been treated. We must show them compassion, charity, and love. Above all, we must not make them feel like strangers. The people of God at all times and in all places are people to accept and welcome strangers. As we reflect on the ministry of Jesus, a constant dynamic was his hospitable movement between being a guest and being a host. Jesus spent time with rich and powerful people and rulers, but he also spent much time with those strangers whom society rejected, marginalized, and refused to relate with. To these, he offered hospitality and welcome. There is a strong tradition in Christianity that seeks to emulate this aspect of

Jesus ministry. As the Apostle Paul exhorts, "When God's people are in need, be ready to help them. Always be eager to practice hospitality." In Romans 12:13, hospitality means "stranger-loving."[254]

To practice hospitality, then, is to learn how to love the stranger. This tradition could offer an important starting point for the shaping of community that can see and respond to dementia in new ways. The question then becomes different: Does the tradition of offering hospitality to strangers provide an adequate model for finding room within Christian communities for people with dementia and those close to them?

The Problem with Being a Stranger

In a sense, the lives of people with dementia could be construed as modern day *gerim*. What problems could arise with equating the people with dementia and their caregivers with *gerim* and the idea of offering hospitality to them as "strangers"? The *gerim* really were strangers. Because they did not come from the same communities, they never could become true-born Israelites; they were forever different. People with dementia are not strangers in such a territorial and ethnic sense, but they are very much part of us. Their status within our communities has not changed. They might change but they will not become strangers. Likewise, the sense of strangerhood that caregivers experience does not mean that they are actually strangers—only that the experience of caring for persons with dementia has made them feel like strangers.

God welcomes the stranger, the disabled, those whom society has pushed to the side. God repositions them from the margins of human caring to the center of divine love. This is a valuable counter to the many forms of malicious social psychology. Thus, Jesus' command to not allow the *gerim* to feel like strangers is directly relevant to those afflicted with dementia.

The Church as Strangers

In an anonymous Letter to Diognetus, a first century apologist reflects on what is different about Christians:

For Christians cannot be distinguished from the rest of human race by country or language or customs. They do not live in cities of their own; they do not use a peculiar form of speech . . . as each man's lot has been cast, and follow the customs of the country in clothing and food and other matters of daily living . . . They live in their own countries, but only as aliens.[255]

This is quite a striking passage. It not only points to the radically different way of life that the early Christians lived, but it shows clearly what their status was in the world:

They share in everything as citizens and endure everything as foreigners. Every foreign land is their fatherland, and yet for them every fatherland is a foreign land. . . . They obey the established laws, but in their own lives they go far beyond what the laws require. They love all men, and by all men they are persecuted.[256]

The vocation of Christians is to live as foreigners in a world within which they have no true home, as their true home is in heaven. As the apostle Peter put it,

Dearly beloved, I beseech you as strangers and pilgrims, abstain from fleshly lusts, which against the soul; Having your conversation honest among the Gentiles: that, whereas they speak against you as evildoers, they may by your good works, which they shall behold, glorify God in the day of visitation. (1 Pet. 2:11–12, KJV)

The vocation of Christians is to live lives that change and transform the world without themselves being polluted by the values, perspectives, and assumptions of the world—to live among people but not to become like them. In other words, *to be a Christian is to live as a stranger.* The vocation of Christians today is to become strangers, or perhaps more accurately, to become a community of strangers. Understood in this way, *the gerim are the church as it exists in the world.* Identifying the church as *gerim* reflects and stems from Jesus' own status as *gerim.* As Cohen puts it:

> The early Church perhaps . . . thought of Jesus as *ger.* Matthew's story of the escape into Egypt (Matt. 2:13–23), linking with Hosea 11:1, makes Jesus clearly a *ger* in Egypt. Luke's story of birth of Jesus contains within it the notion that Jesus was a stranger who found lodgings in a manger. When this can be linked with Jeremiah 14:8—"Why are you like an alien in the land, like a traveler who stays in lodgings?"—the picture becomes clear.[257]

Jesus is *ger,* the ultimate stranger. Significantly, the early church identified itself as *paroikos,* the Greek equivalent of *ger:*[258]

> The church was the new Israel, was therefore a nation of sojourners who lived as citizens of God's household. They were not in the world but lived in it. The people of God were *gerim* who are protected by God. Whether in their ancient or recent history. In Jesus, the people knew God to be *ger,* with whom they shared a soul.[259]

Thus, strangerhood and being a Christian can be seen to be one and the same thing. To follow Jesus the *ger,* is to be a disciple. *Gerim* make up the community of God; we are strangers who are called to welcome strangers. Thus, it may be slightly inaccurate to suggest that the best frame for the church's attitude toward those affected by dementia is the church's key vocation of offering hospitality to strangers. It might be more appropriate to suggest that the church is called to offer hospitality among strangers. The difference is subtle but important.

Hospitality among Strangers

In Matthew 25, Jesus offers a picture of the final judgment. In this breathtaking apocalypse, there is terrifying separation between the good (the sheep, the faithful) and the evil (the goats, the unfaithful). The criterion appears to be not only what people believed, but also the manners in which they put their beliefs into action. Salvation also becomes a criterion for those who will be invited into the kingdom. To those who only offered food, water, visitation, presence, and hospitality to those who were in need, Jesus' response is stunning—in ministering to people in such ways, they have been ministering to God. In v. 35, Jesus says, "[When] I was a stranger and you invited me in." The thing to notice here is the transformation that occurred between what Jesus was and what he became. He was invited in and welcomed. Paradoxically, he no longer was a stranger when he was held within the community of strangers.

This is an important observation regarding to how the church might go about re-describing the ways in which it should respond to people with dementia and those who seek to offer them love and care. The pattern of the Gospel reveals that Jesus, not unlike people with dementia, was clearly perceived as a stranger by the society around him, even though he in fact was one of them (John 1:46). People's simple act of inviting Jesus in was a profound movement away from his socially ascribed role as "the stranger" and toward a repositioning of him as someone worthy of the offer of hospitality. To estrange the outsider is to make God a stranger. The object of extending hospitality to strangers is to stop perceiving them as strangers, not just offering them welcome. The intention is not to continually minister to people with dementia as if they remain forever strangers and empower their status as friends. Ministering to people with dementia has the end goal of revealing that they are not in fact strangers at all.

The idea of offering hospitality to strangers, in the sense of caring for people outside of the Christian community, remains pivotal. When it comes to Christians who have dementia, however, the welcoming of strangers requires a parallel dynamic that focuses on hospitality between and among them. Hospitality between strangers begins with the assumption that people with dementia are irrevocably members of the community of strangers. Such hospitality does not have to invite them in at all, as they already are fully present, but it does need to find them and recognize their existence. Malcomb Goldsmith makes this point well:

> I look back with shame on my five years as a rector of a busy church in the center of an England city some twenty years ago. I don't think I can recall meeting a single person with dementia during that period. If you don't look for them and if you are not ready to welcome and accept them, then they easily go to church elsewhere and invariably becomes nowhere and we are all impoverished as a result.[260]

Clearly, the ongoing welcoming of people with dementia and those who care for them is not always available, or at least it does not always feel like it is available. In church, the act of welcoming people with dementia and their families has to be central to the strategies of mission, evangelism, worship, and pastoral care.

A Theology of Welcome and Belonging

The key is to create places of belonging where people with dementia and those who offer care and support to them can find "space" that is truly theirs and within which they can express the full experience of dementia—its pain, its affliction, and its lament as well as its joy and possibilities. Dementia is as much a relational and spiritual condition as it is neurological. It is overcoming malicious social psychology and negative theological positioning that requires particular forms of personal relationships that make welcoming, belonging, and truly being in the moment with others a possibility. Lean Vanier stresses its impact:

> The basic human need is for at least one person who believes and trusts in us. But it is not enough . . . Each of us needs to belong, not just to one person but to a family, friends, a group, and a culture.[261]

Tragically, the ways in which people with dementia and their caregivers are framed and treated by society often functions in precisely the opposite way. Rather than drawing people into community, they throw them into the role of strangers and destroy any sense of belonging for both the sufferers and those around them. Vanier says, "We do not discover who we are, we do not reach true humanness in a solitary state; it through mutual dependency, in weakness, in learning through belonging."[262] In order to be remembered well now and in the future, we must recognize how crucial it is to create spaces of "belonging," which is different from simply "being included." Everyone needs to belong and be present somewhere, wherever that is. Everyone needs to be missed if they are not present in the place where they belong. In order to belong in the community of strangers, people with dementia and their families need to be missed when they are absent. Otherwise, they do not belong, and there is no true community for them.

The theological framework makes it clear that creating such spaces of belonging is not an option for the church. Rather, it is an act of faithfulness and a living out of its true humanity on which church can reflect regarding their own and collective experiences of people with dementia. Are they missed when they are not there, or are they there but also being missed?

A Theology of Visitation

Learning how to miss people involved with dementia requires knowing that they are "there" in the first place, that the church not only includes people with dementia and their caregivers, but also takes time to be with them, get to know them, and show them love. So we need to visit them to overcome our estrangement and begin to redescribe and relearn to love one another, in the power of Spirit, in ways that are constructive and healing.

The term "visit" in Latin means "to see, notice, or observe" (hence the word "video"). Clearly, there is a tendency not to see people with dementia properly. This, in effect, is the essence of malicious social psychology. To visit someone properly requires learning to be with them physically and to see them in the right ways. To learn to rethink dementia in fundamental ways requires learning the practice of *visitation*. As we visit one another, we learn what it means to offer and to receive hospitality among strangers.

Visitation has three dimensions to it: 1) Negatively, it can relate to forms of suffering or disaster that are visited upon individuals or communities—often by God. Such visitation can be punishment for sins or the infliction of illness. 2) It relates to the creative appearance of God as he reaches into creation to minister his people. God's visitations are profound and deep and designed to initiate change and transformation. When God comes to visit someone, he does so for a purpose, and that purpose is always revelatory and transformative. The visitation is both temporary (Jesus' earthly ministry) and permanent (through the power of Holy Spirit). 3) It relates to Jesus' statement from Matthew's passage (Math. 25:35–36). So we who visit can encounter God in the sensitivity of our touch, our words, and a gentle presence that transcends all of time. *Visitation is the embodiment of God's actions toward creation. As we visit those with dementia and those who care for them, so we bring God with us.*

Visiting the sick is thus seen to be a deeply theological Christian practice and crucial way of offering hospitality among strangers. It is the simple but radical practice of visiting. Theology makes sense only when it is practiced. If someone visits the "wrong person," then their presence will not be healing.

Rethinking the Gesture of Love

We love people because of the pleasure we get from their having certain capacities (response and reaction). It is not 100% accurate, but capacity does not define our humanness, yet it matters. In fact, this is evident to those among us who are close to people with dementia. It matters because now they no longer can remember or communicate with us. It matters that we also feel that we are losing them in fundamental ways. It matters that we sometimes do not feel the same about them as we did when they were fit, healthy, and unafflicted. Capacities may not define people, but they do have an impact on their relationships. Capacities are not the criteria for love, but they do inhibit its expression.

If we can have a choice to love or to stop to love someone in a certain way, that it may possibly lead to a healthier and more helpful manner. But it is not adequate to suggest that we stop loving a person, even if that in fact is possible. We cannot say, "It's not good that you exist, or "It's not good that you're in this world," which are the correct responses to our loved ones encountering with people who have dementia. In fact, we feel precisely that way many times. The manifestations of love are many and varied, and many of the ways in which we normally assume love to be expressed are challenged by those who see and experience the world of love differently through the experience of dementia, or when it comes to the expression of love in the context of advanced dementia. We have to think about the gesture of love. We will have to let go of some of the old ways in which we loved the person. We need to let go the old ways and accept that things have changed and that the old modes of love are different and learn to love through ones gestures, presence, and touch and movement. Our act of faith is to hold on to people as they develop and change through the disease process and to learn what it means to be with them and to love the emerging person. This will be painful, alienating, and difficult, but the cross of Jesus reveals to us that often love is precisely this way. We may have to learn to see (new) love differently and to realize that different forms of love can be valid and totally justified.

The new forms of love may be quite different, and although we can grow into them, they are filled with both sorrow and joy. It is absolutely crucial, however, to remember that love remains love so even if its shape shifts and changes. Caring for the bodily needs is a deep expression of love, but it is not the same as sharing in someone's emotional life, planning together for the future, or sharing dreams. This love may not be romantic as such, but it is more than just feeling—it is a way of being in the world. Sometimes, it is hard, willful, intentional, and deeply disappointment. This is often profoundly the case we are faced with regarding the losses that accompany Alzheimer's. But if we can recognize the way that we love remains real, even if it has to adapt to the rhythm of the disease process, we need not feel guilty when our feelings shift, change, and oscillate. Free in this way, we just might be able to discover new and hopeful ways to love as the old and tested ways move on. Such a process may begin with weeping as it is pointed out in the meditation of Psalm 88.

With a sincere, heartfelt prayer and hope, may this material offer positive, hopeful, and realistic places to begin to rethink the practices of love within the context of Alzheimer's. There is much room for hope and joy to run alongside grief and lament—that is the nature of love.

10

Memory and Divine Embrace

"I will not forget you! See, I have engraved you on the palms of my hands." (Isaiah 49:15–16)

There is nothing about dementia that can destroy the personhood or humanness of the individual with dementia, nor is there anything that can taint a person's unending being lovable. This is not to try to romanticize dementia; it is simply to offer a different description that will frame it in such a way that we can see people as persons and recognize that dementia is but another example of the limitedness and mortality of the human condition. This way we have retaken some of the territory that rightly belongs to theology and pastoral care. To redescribe dementia, personhood, and humanness brings us to an important issue in relation to dementia—the issue of memory.

Dementia is a journey. There is a real sense in which the experience of dementia itself can be viewed as a journey—that is, a profound movement from one way of being in the world to a quite different way of encountering ourselves and others. Each step along the journey brings with it different needs, opportunities, and challenges. During the later stage of journey, the time in the process of moving into dementia, when people begin to lose certain things that previously they assumed to be central for their sense of identity, one of the most primary among these is their memory. It is the loss of memory that is perhaps the most feared aspect of dementia. Who are we when we have forgotten ourselves and those whom we once loved? Who are we before God when we have forgotten who God is? For many people, the idea of losing their memory evokes a deep fear of losing themselves. Not to remember is to cease to exist.

The Fear of Dementia

There can be no greater fear than the possibility of losing memory. Modernity may have offered us longevity but at some threat to our human wellbeing. From James Woodward, "Dementia poses many fundamental theological and pastoral challenges."[263] According to Albert Jewell, "The big issues raised by dementia; personhood and identity, mind and memory, body and soul and the value to be found in every human life, prepare ones for a challenge."[264]

Dementia is more feared than cancer. In the U.K., their YouGo poll of 2,000 people on the behalf of Alzheimer's Research yielded these results:

1. 31% fear dementia the most, 27% fear cancer the most, and 18% fear death the most.
2. Dementia fears extend to all ages. 52% of U.K. adults from age 30 to 50 fear their parents will develop dementia. This is compared to 42% most afraid of cancer, and 33% most afraid of heart attacks.
3. Among retirees, 34% worry about health the most, compared to 33% who worry about things such as money. Specifically, 52% worry about dementia, 33% cancer, and 39% stroke.
4. Regarding the difference between *concern* and *fear*, cancer exceeds dementia—35% versus 24% are concerned than fearful of contracting cancer.[265]

In sum, cancer evoke concern; dementia evokes fear. At the heart of people's fear is the fear of losing their memory, and in so doing losing themselves. According to different stories told, the experience of advanced dementia seems like the end of everything—the end of identity, the end of one's humanness. Almost all of the things that liberal cultures assume to be valuable in a human being appear to be taken away from the person in the later stages of dementia. If losing our memory and our ability to reason and respond at an intellectual level means losing our humanness, then who would not be afraid? Is dementia not worthy of fear—an illness that seems to bring about death before it actually occurs? As has be shown, the fear of dementia is closely tied to the prevailing secular cultural worldview, which runs counter to that of the Christian faith.

Tragedy and Possibility

While reasons abound to be hopeful within the church, those who claim to be participants in God's church are also participants in the surrounding culture, and they tend to fear the same things as others do for the same reasons. When those fears are transferred uncritically into one's theology and practice, however, things become complicated. In a religious culture, where remembering the acts of God and proclaiming the name of Jesus are often assumed to be central to salvation, a loss that prevents someone from engaging in such intellectually oriented, propositional, spiritual activities creates dissonance and uncertainty. While it might not be articulated often, fear run like a silent undertow through the framing of and the responses to many experiences of advanced dementia. The deep forgetfulness and often profound changes to personality and perceived identity that accompany dementia raise theological questions: As a demented person, are we still saved, even though we have forgotten Jesus? Who will we be in heaven if we have changed so drastically in the present?" How can we love God when we have forgotten who God is? How can we be us when we no longer know who we are? If our hope lies in the resurrection, which person will be resurrected—the pre-dementia one or the current one? Such theological questions have crucial practical significance, and the answers will determine how we conceptualize, understand, and respond to people with dementia.

In advanced dementia, a person's memory problem becomes severe, and eventually the person become totally dependent on others for most or all of their needs. At this stage, many of the difficult philosophical, theological, and practical questions that we have looked at come into sharp focus. To focus on advanced dementia is not to suggest that other places along the journey are less important. The fear after the diagnosis, the steady decline and gradual loss of memory, the feeling that one is losing everything that one loves and feels worthwhile—these are terrible experiences for those with dementia and for those who love them and desire to offer care and support. Dementia is a special affliction—it is a journey into a progressive form of disease, which inevitably is shaped not only by what is happening at the moment, but also by the fear and uncertainty of what will happen in the future. By focusing on the later stages of the journey, it will make the traveling a little easier for those who are just beginning. Dementia is an extremely difficult condition to live with, both for sufferers and for those who care for them. Suffering is a key dimension of the experience of dementia for those who bear the weight of the condition and for those who care for them. Dementia is not a romantic disease; nevertheless, it need not be defined only as suffering. There is room for hope.

Dementia: A Problem of Memory

The standard story of dementia and its relationship with memory goes something beyond like this: The most prominent features of dementia are the ways in which it takes away one's memories. Dementia is a condition that is marked by, among other things, a profound loss of memory caused by damage to the particular areas of the brain that are responsible for memory. Because memories are crucial for a human being's sense of self, major memory loss inevitably leads to a crisis or even a loss of identity. If we cannot remember who we are, how can we know who we are? How can we be ourselves when we have no idea who we are? Thus, we are our memories. Filmmaker Luis Bunuel believes this:

> You have to begin to lose your memory, if only in bits
> and pieces, to realize that memory is what makes our
> lives. Life without memory is no life at all, just as an

intelligence without the possibility of expression is not really an intelligence. Our memory is our coherence, our reason, our feeling, even our action. Without it, we are nothing.[266]

Bunuel's statement seems quite logical and his thinking represents the results of the British YouGov poll. How does he know, however, since he has never had the experience of dementia, and on what basis did he come to such a firm conclusion as, "Life without memory is no life at all." By description, none of us can express what it is like to live without memory. Presumably, Bunuel is projecting what he imagines it would be like to have no memory. Projection and imagining, however, are not always accurate representations of actual experience. Bunuel's perspective is probably understandable in the light of society's general fears that surround dementia. Surprisingly, similar thinking is reflected in David Keck's theological account of memory and selfhood when he describes Alzheimer's disease as "deconstruction- incarnate":

> It becomes possible to say that Alzheimer's disease represents deconstruction incarnate. The instability of meaning and free play of signifiers which deconstructionists enjoy talking about become manifest most clearly in an Alzheimer's patient. Particularly in the latter stages, the slipperiness of a patient's language becomes apparent.[267]

For Keck, the idea of deconstruction seems to relate to the slipping away of the structures of meaning that sustain persons with dementia as the persons they previously were. As language slips away, so do persons as they were previously known.[268] At the heart of the de-constructive process is the loss of memory, as Keck asserts,

> It is impossible to distinguish between ourselves and our memories.... *We are our memories*, and without them we have but a physical resemblance to that person we each

suppose ourselves to be . . . The apparent dissolution
of the mnemonic capacities . . . raises most serious and
profound questions about human existence.[269]

Like Bunuel, Keck seems to assume that human beings essentially
are their memories. The perspectives of Bunuel and Keck at first seems
to make some sense. It seems "natural" to associate ourselves—what we
are as unique, self-aware individuals—with what we can remember about
ourselves. As Buber and Kitwood have made clear, however, the distance
one stands from the object of one's interest matters. Assumptions about
the centrality of memory for determining selfhood become deeply
problematic from the perspective of people experiencing dementia.
Christine Bryden, a woman going through the experience of pre-senile
dementia, makes this point well:

> Dementia has been called the "theological disease" by
> David Keck, who cared for his mother with AD. There is
> prolonged mental deterioration, and no presumption of
> the existence of a cognitive person theologically. He said
> the loss of "memory entails a loss of self." And the apparent
> disintegration of a human being. Perhaps AD patients
> can remind us that death and loss of control belong at the
> heart of theological reflection. David Keck's views shock
> me as a person with dementia in the early stages. Can
> I truly regard dementia as "deconstruction incarnate,"
> "disintegrative, non-redemptive . . . amoral"? Certainly,
> I challenge the view of AD International that the "mind
> is absent and the body an empty shell." The question is,
> where does this journey begin, and at what stage can you
> deny me my selfhood and my spirituality?[270]

Similar to the reason that the medical model of dementia is difficult
for those with dementia, so are certain theological/philosophical
formulations of their experiences. Bryden's concern about Keck's
proposition is a powerful reminder that clever theological language and

academic conceptualizations of human experiences, even when intended for compassionate ends, may not look quite so cleaver or compassionate when they are read by those who are experiencing "the concept." Such malicious spiritual positioning inevitably is unhelpful and destructive. For Bryden, the statement that "life without memory is no life at all" is simply wrong—there is more to being human than memory alone. The changes in her life may be profound, but the key for her is to find new ways of encountering God when the old ways have faded and disappeared:

> I believe that I am much more than just my brain structure and function, which is declining daily. My creation in the divine image is as a soul capable of love, sacrifice, and hope, not as a perfect human being, in mind or body. I want you to relate to me in that way, seeing me as God sees me. I am confident that even if the continuous damage to my temporal lobe might diminish the intensity of my God-experience, there will be other ways in which I can maintain my relationship with God.[271]

She answers the question, "Will she know God when she can no longer remember?" in this way:

> David Keck reflects on the importance of the memory of God's past deeds to the Israelites, and yet Christian confession and creed start with the words "I believe," not "I remember." Will I know before God if I can no longer remember? . . . As I unfold before God, as this disease unwraps me, opening up the treasures of what lies within my multifold personality, I can feel safe as each layer is gently opened out. God's everlasting arms will be beneath me, upholding me. "I will trust in God," who will hold me safe in his memory, until that glorious day of Resurrection, when each facet of my personality can be expressed to the full.[272]

Such a description of the dementia experience could not be further away from the idea of "deconstruction incarnate" or "memory is all that we are." Bryden recognizes that her memory and her cognitive faculties are slipping away, but she frames that slippage quite differently. She trusts that God will remember her. When her journey has ended, her true self will continue to exist and ultimately even flourish in the resurrection. "Who she is" is held and sustained within the memories of God, and that is where she finds her hope and her strength.

Being Remembered by God

In an old English hymn, "According to Thy Gracious Word," all the verses but the last, "when thou shalt in thy kingdom come, Jesus, remember me," focus on our remembering Jesus because of his command to remember him eucharistically; but the last verse lays a task of remembering back with God, on our behalf. Imaging where in the midst of deeply forgetful people, who clearly have been forgotten, and discovering a key that unlocks aspects of their memories that were otherwise inaccessible, we need to recognize something deeply powerful in the hymn that calls us to remember while we can, but to trust that God will remember for us when we cannot.

The idea of being remembered by God is a frequent theme in pastoral literature, and while not uncontested,[273] it has potential for helping us understand some vital but often hidden aspects of memory loss in dementia. The following story opens up this way of thinking quite helpfully:

> An elderly lady with dementia paced the corridors of a nursing home restlessly, and repeating over and over just one word. . . . The staff, in fact, were at a loss to understand the reason for her stress. The word she repeated was "God." . . . One day, a nurse walked alongside with her, up and down the corridor. Suddenly, in a flash of inspiration, the nurse asked the lady, "Are you afraid

that you will forget God?" The elderly lady answered emphatically, "Yes, Yes!" The nurse was able to say to her, "You know even if you should forget God, He will not forget you. He has promised that." . . . The assurance was what the elderly lady needed to hear. She quickly became more peaceful, and that strange behavior ceased. She was responding positively to care which extended beyond the needs of body and mind—care of the human spirit.[274]

This moving story, ending the woman's fears in a situation where she did not understand the deepest things that were so important to her is a frightening thought. It is both touching and disturbing to know that what was always been central to her life—"God"—was slipping away and that she felt that she could express her distress only through bodily movements that were open to multiple interpretations. The key that unlocked this woman's distress came from someone who saw beyond the "obvious" interpretation of her situation based on the normal associations that come with her diagnosis, and asked a simple but profound question, "Are you afraid that you will forget God?" The deep fear of forgetting is overcome by the deeper promise of being remembered. This reminds of the plea of one of the thieves who was hung alongside Jesus on the cross, "Remember me when you come into your kingdom" (Luke 23:42). The woman's walking in the corridor was a way of seeking the same thing. The response came in a compassionate act of spiritual listening that reinforced God's promise, "Never will I leave you; never will I forsake you" (Heb. 13:5). This assurance of God's remembrance helped her to become peaceful.

Our hope lies in the fact that we exist because God sustains us, and because of that we are living in the memories of God. As long as God remembers us, who we are will remain: "I will not forget you, See, I have engraved you on the palms of my hands" (Isa. 49:15–16). This resonates with Kitwood's suggestion that we are sustained and identified as persons through our relationships with others—except that here, it is God who ultimately is responsible for holding onto us and remembering us well.

Kitwood wants carers to engage in memorial practices without transcendence. Caregivers can be not only givers of care but bestowals of a kind of immorality by recalling for others around them what the person with Alzheimer's disease no longer can recall in order to strengthen the remembering of that person and to keep his or her role in the story of the community alive in the corporate memory.[275]

When others forget us, God always remembers. Again, Steve Sapp puts in this way:

It is also possible to speak of God's memory in this light. Whether the individual [or] the Western religious tradition certainly affirms that God remembers. Some comfort, therefore, can be found in the fact that God's memory is unfailing, even if that of any given human being is defective or even totally lost. God never forgets.[276]

We can, and should, mourn someone's personal loss of memory, but if God remembers us, we are provided with a source of deep and enduring hope. We are not what we remember; we are remembered because we are God's, the one who cannot forget us. Memory is first and foremost something that is done for us, rather than something we achieve on our own.

The Problem with God's Memory

As useful and comforting as the idea may be of the memory of God providing a hopeful future for people with profound memory loss, it may not be as helpful as it first appears. Peter Kevern presents a typology of four models to conceptualize the role of memory:

- A "Traditional/Historical" model, in which memory is central to placing the individual in a shared tradition.

- An "Open to God" model, which envisages each individual as being moved by the Spirit into an ever-richer enjoyment of God's fellowship.
- A "Growth" model, which envisages the individual as continuously journeying toward full spiritual maturity.
- A "Remembered by God" model, which Goldsmith takes to be the "only theological model which seems to encapsulate the 'Good News' for the person with dementia," stressing that people are remembered by God long before and long after they make any recognizable response to God.[277]

While Kevern acknowledges that the "remembered by God" approach has some pastoral utility, on deeper reflection, he finds reason to view it with some concern:

> This simplicity may be the reason why the slogan "God never forgets" seems to crop up repeatedly in the literature.[278]

> [T]he model has its limitations both as a theological and a pastoral strategy. First, there is a tendency to denial of the depth of the question raised (although people forget, God always remembers) and a profound pessimism (dementia is understood only as loss and as a step toward death). There is no continuing "presence" of God in dementia, but only the eschatological and somewhat vague hope that God will make everything all right in the end. Amidst the abandonments and bereavements of dementia, the person is abandoned by and bereaved of the living God.[279]

For Kevern, the idea of being remembered by God is framed in some of the literature, but there is tendency to see that remembrance as prospective and primarily eschatological in nature. He perceives that the assumption tends to be that God will remember in the future, rather than that God remembers in the present. For now, God remains absent and impassive in a sense, waiting for the time when his memory will come to fulfillment. Meanwhile, persons with dementia are left alone in their suffering and concern. They can have hope that God is not going to forget them, but they have little to give them hope that God is with them in the present, sharing in their sufferings. Kevern concludes that the idea of being remembered by God requires more theological capital than it is worth:

> We may conclude, therefore, that the proclamation of a God who always remembers, however comforting, comes at too high a theological cost: it leaves us alone in our struggle with the terrifying contingency and flux of dementia. maintaining hope only in a God who will somehow be there at the end of it all. It places God on the outside of the process of change and deterioration, uninvolved in the messy business of living and dying in dementia; waiting at the door, as it were, for it all to be over and the victim to be released into death.[280]

Kevern has a point with regard to those who develop the idea of God remembering from an understanding of God that perceives him as distant and impassible.[281] Even in the more developed theological work on dementia, there is a tendency to hold onto God as, "uncompromisingly impassable and sovereign, outside of and above the situation, not within it." If we formulate hope for people with dementia as existing only in the future, then indeed there is a danger that we implicitly abandon them in the present. If the memory of God sustaining hope only for a possible future without being active in the present, it remains hopeful, but not necessary all that helpful. Kevern goes on to develop an image of God as intimately and deeply involved with the suffering of creation, a perspective that clearly is more advanced than models of remembering based on God's future presence.

Kevern is correct with regard to the dangers of creating an image of God that is distant and impassive. The scripture account of God is of a person who is deeply involved with creation and who suffers with people rather than distancing himself from them. The incarnation, cross, and resurrection of Jesus indicate that God is deeply implicated in both suffering and the joy of human existence and the world. As Dietrich Bonhoeffer put it, "Only the suffering God can help."[282] If God is perceived as distant and impassive, and his memory functions only in the future, then his involvement in the present is limited to his passive role as sustainer, with suffering belonging only to the collective experience of his creation. It is difficult to equate such an image with the scriptures that stress "God is Love" (e.g., 1 Jn 4:8). Love that truly loves is inevitably open to suffering and rejection. Any theological framework that omits this crucial dynamic falls short of perceiving the glory of God's love, and in so doing makes it possible for God to be seen an abandoning people with dementia in the present.

The problem with Kevern's position that we are held and sustained by the memory of God is his suggestion that the idea of being remembered by God necessarily places God outside of the situation of people with dementia. It may be true that some approaches do this, but those who do are overlooking the significance of Jesus' words in Matthew 28:20, "and surely I will be with you always, to the very end of the age." Jesus does not say that he will be with his people only or even primarily at some point in the future. His clear statement is that he will be with us both in the present and the future. If God is truly with us, then his memory cannot simply be something that becomes active in, or is even primarily oriented toward, the future. God may remember in the future, but God also remembers the past and the future simultaneously in the present. The point is that to reject the idea of God's remembering on the grounds that it ignores the present is to misunderstand the nature of memory in general and God's memory in particular. To misunderstand the nature and purpose of God's memory is to misunderstand the practices of God in the lives of people with dementia.

What Does It Mean to Remember?

To understand the importance of God's memory as it impacts our understanding of dementia, we need to begin by reflecting on what it actually means to remember anything at all. Of course, human memory is not the same as God's memory; nonetheless, in order to understand something of God's memory, we need to understand the way in which human memory functions. It is only as we come to understand the strangeness and complexity of human memory that we can understand the significance of being remembered by God.

On the surface, human memory seems to be quite straightforward. It has to do with the ways in which the brain captures, records, processes, and retains information that it gathers through experience. When we see and experience something, the brain records it, and we can "play it back" later when the memory is required. Short-term memory refers to experiences and information that we have encountered in recent experiences. Long-term memory refers to things that have occurred in the more distant past. The past informs our sense of the present, and the present informs our understandings of the past. Together, the past and present together inform our perceptions of what the future might look like. It is in the constant, ongoing movement between our short- and long-term memories that we are able to orient ourselves in ways that allow us to gain a sense of continuity and flow through time.

This is the kind of understanding of memory that we encounter in St. Augustine's formulation of memory in his classic book series, *Confessions*. For him, memory is basically an archive of images and experiences that a person accumulates over time—"like a great field or a spacious palace," or a "storehouse for countless images."[283] The storehouse is a private place that resides within the individual, "an inner place."[284] Augustine also sees memory as a capacity that humans use to store and retrieve information. He equates the memory with the mind and the self:

> But the mind and memory are one and the same. We
> even call the memory the mind, for when we tell another
> to remember something we say "bear this in mind," and

when we forget something we say "it was not in my mind," or "it slipped in my mind."... Yet I do not understand the power of memory that is in myself, although without it I could not even speak of myself. The power of memory is great, O Lord. It is awe-inspiring in its profound and incalculable complexity. Yet it is my mind: it is myself.[285]

In this understanding, memory is a cognitive and intellectual capacity that resides purely within the mind of an individual. In fact, memory is mind, and inevitably, memory also is the self. Our essential selves, our personal identities are tied to what we can remember. If this the case, then the suggestion that "Life without memory is no life at ball" make perfect sense. As logical as this may sound, it is not the way in which memory functions.

What Do We Actually Remember?

Memory is not like the simple see-record-store-playback model above—it is much more complex. It is more than simply "retrieving different kinds of information: there is also a conviction that this episode is part of our personal history, related to events that came before and have occurred since."[286] Memory is the product of both biography and history and not simply recalling things in an nonedited, noninterpreted manner. We read our memories through our emotions and our ongoing biographies. The information that we gather in the past is important for us as we encounter the present; however, not all of the information that we use to form our memories emerges from direct recall. As Daniel Schachet, a Harvard professor of psychology, observes,

We are constantly making use of information acquired in the past. In order to type these sentences into my computer, I must retrieve words and grammatical rules that I learned long ago, yet I do not have any subjective experience of "remembering" them. Every time you start your car and begin to drive, you are calling on knowledge and skills you acquired years earlier, but you do not feel as though you are revisiting the past.[287]

Memory work at different levels and utilizes a variety of different aspects of the brain. The brain has a series of memory systems that it uses to process the past in different ways:

1. Semantic Memory relates to how we remember concepts and facts.
2. Procedural Memory relates to remembering how to do things. It is that aspect of memory that enables us to develop the skills and habits that allow us to engage in certain tasks and procedures.... But someone could still play intricate melodies on the piano even if, arguably, the kind of meaning that was associated it with earlier in life didn't appear to be present.[288]
3. Episodic Memory relates to the "subjective experience of explicitly remembering past incidents." To be experience as memory, the retrieved information must be recollected in the context of a particular time and place and with some reference to oneself as a participant in the episode.[289]
4. Psychologist Endel Tulving draws out the implications of this point: The particular state of consciousness that characterizes the experience of remembering includes the rememberer's belief that the memory is a more or less true replica of the original event, even if only a fragmented and hazy one, as well as the belief that the event is part of his own past. Remembering, for the rememberer, is mental time travel, a sort of reliving of something that happened in the past.[290]

Memory in its episodic form is a creative act of fact, faith, and imagination. Our memory is the place where, in varied and diverse ways, our history is stored. Who we are and from where we have come forth, where we are now and what we hope for in the future—are inevitably tied up with our ability to remember. True, certain procedural memories will function without the memory of our history or sense of who we are, but if our episodic memory is taken from us, if we cannot process the past and find meaning and understanding of who we are in the present, then it at least appears to be difficult to see in what sense we are the people we were before. This is what Bunuel and Keck are pointing toward.

Dementia in all of its different forms leads ultimately to a profound loss of episodic memory. If we assume that memory is equal to identity, then the loss of this aspect of our memory inevitably will be perceived as leading to a loss of self and self-identity. Memory understood in this way raises profound questions. What it is that gives us continuity of identity? What is the connection between what we were when we were remembering and what we are not now that we have forgotten what we were? These are more than just questions about personal identity in a psychological sense. Theologically, such questions raise complex issues, such as precisely which "me" will be resurrected? The "me" that I can remember, or the "me" that I am now. As we live our lives in what, for some, is perceived as clearly an eternal present, what was may have no obvious connection with what is. The answer "God will remember you" indeed is powerful and attractive, given the understanding of memory currently discussed and the significance of episodic memory in particular. If God remembers us, then our "vanishing self" in some sense will be preserved.

This raises the question, however, of precisely what it is that we think we would like to have preserved. What might one mean by "preserved?" In order for something to be preserved, we need first to assume that we know and understand the "thing" that need preserving; otherwise, we would never know if it was or was not preserved. Put slightly differently, if we are concerned about "ourself" being in some way preserved, we needs to have some sense of what or who "ourself" actually is. Likewise, if we are worried about losing "ourselves," then we presumably think that we know who we are, which of course takes us back to Bonhoeffer's question, which opened this book, "Who am I?"

What are Memories and What Are they Made of?

Clearly, memory is not quite as straightforward as it appears to be. Our memories are formed according to what we see and remember, but the remembered past is much more fragile, deceptive, and mysterious than we presume. Therefore, memory is not simply a straightforward collection of what has happened in the past. We are deeply involved in the creation of our memories, which do not function the way that computer retrieval systems or tape recorders do. With both examples, what one puts in is what one gets out. The quality may vary, but the content and meaning are more or less the same. Memory is different. Memory is as subjective as it is objective. Memories are constructed not only out of what we think we remember in an historical sense, but also in accordance with our current needs, desires, and the ways we see the world and expect it to be. Memories are also saturated with feeling and emotions. When we remember something, we often feel it emotionally. But the emotion we attach to the memory are not necessarily representative of the emotion we felt when we originally created that memory. It will more than likely relate more closely to our current emotional state and the way in which that memory has gathered meaning and feeling over time. Memories are also intertwined not only with other memories, but with the rememberer's memories of the memories. In 2018, I was struggling to remember what happened at a group picnic that I had attended in 2012, when suddenly the memory came to me. Therefore, the next time I try to remember the party, I will not go back to the original memory but will go back to the last time I remembered it and re-remember the memory and how I felt about it when I remembered it in 2018. In other words, when we remember something, we do not simple go back to the original memory; rather, we remember the memory as it came to us the last time ones remembered it. So I remember the last time I remembered the event, rather than simply remembering the original event. This is one reason why the feelings and experiences around memories can shift and change.

Schachter suggests that memories might be better framed as collages or jigsaw puzzles rather than pictures or tape recordings.[291] Our memories do not record everything, and they do not simply present straightforward historical pictures. Instead, they present us with selective and highly constructed perspectives on what we believe happened. Memory, then, is a highly complex process that cannot be fully explained by reflecting only on the technicalities of neural involvement. Memories are always and inevitably constructions and reconstructions of the past that deeply involve biography, experience, and emotion.

Because of this creative and emotional dimension to memory, the meaning and interpretation of memories can change quite quickly as something occurs that makes people rethink and reconstruct the past. It is obvious that within such a process there is a great deal of room for misinterpretation and distortion. Such distortion can relate to attitudes, moods, or emotional states that deeply affect the ways in which we interpret and understand memory. Distortion may relate to the content of a memory: we assume that something happened that did not actually occur, or we put a different interpretation on an event, the meaning of which we assumed was previously settled. "I feel much better about things today" indicates such a change in the meaning of memories. Or a child might not remember that he had been abused until later in life, when certain things are pointed out making it obvious that his original interpretation of the memory was flawed and/or the way he perceived the experience was misinterpreted.

This perspective on memory is not to suggest that we do not know anything at all about past, or that it is impossible to remember anything accurately. Clearly, we do know some things and remember them quite well. It does indicate the ways in which our past and our memories of the past are much more mysterious, fragile, unclear, and less accurate than we often assume them to be. Indeed, we have forgotten most of what has happened to us in the past, and that is how it should be. To remember everything would be a most unhealthy state. Sometimes we need to forget to survive.[292]

The essential point, to claim that people with dementia have lost their identity because they have forgotten certain things about themselves and the world, is not a straightforward claim. None of us is clear about who we are if who we are is determined by the accuracy of what we can remember. How, then, can we be sure of who we are? Is Bonhoeffer's answer to "Who am I?" plausible?

Living in the Memories of God: A Theology about Memory

Who can understand the human heart but God alone. Human memory inevitably is flawed and open to deception and distortion (Jeremiah 17:7–10). This, combined with our inherent fallenness, means that there is a real sense in which we can never know who we really are. This self-amnesia is a fact the Freud brought out many years ago in his reflections on the human unconscious. It reaches other dimensions when perceived theologically. We may be uncertain about who we are but God is not. God remembers us properly; he remembers us because he knows us (Psalms 139:2–12).

God's knowledge of us is too great to understand. At the heart of God's intimate knowing of human beings lies his remembering us. In Psalms 8:4, the psalmist asks the wistful question of what it is to be a human being: "What is man that you are mindful of him, the son of man that you care for him?" The adjective "mindful" derives from the verb "remember" (Hebrew, *zkr*). While the psalmist may not be totally clear in his mind about what a human being is, he is crystal clear about one thing: God is mindful of human beings. To be human is to be held in the memory of God—he watches over human beings, knows them intimately, and always remembers them.

The Memory of God

Recognizing that human beings may struggle to know who they are but are always held and known by God's memory has important implications. For starters, it means that we need to be careful when we say or believe that persons with advanced dementia have lost their identity because they have lost their memory. Our brief reflections on the psychology of memory have indicated that an over-identification of memory with identity may be deceptive. Theologically, it is not our memory that assures our identity; it is the memory of God and, by proxy, the memory of others. But quite apart from the psychological and theological difficulties in making memory the seat of identity, such a suggestion is dangerous for the practical reasons that have been outlined previously. If we believe that people with dementia have somehow gone or, to use Keck's phrase, if we assume that all is left is "a physical resemblance" to those persons we once knew, then precisely who or what do we think we are dealing with in our personal encounters with people who have advanced dementia?

If someone is not the persons they used to be, then who are they? If we do not know who they are, then how and why might we desire to care for them? As Peter Singer points out, the sufferers have lost all sense of identity over time; they have lost their personhood, and therefore they have the right of moral protection.[293] As we have seen, the suggestion that a person has gone and all that is left is a physical resemblance, even in the most advanced stages of dementia, is simply wrong. Certainly, the person may have changed, and all aspects of what we and the person thought they were will become different, sometimes quite radically so. Maybe the person does not recognize ones, and perhaps they struggle to recognize him; nevertheless, the person's identity—that which holds him in his place of self and humanness—is not lost or forgotten. The tension between what we see and experience as we encounter the person who has clearly been changed by dementia and the suggestion that his identity remains held in the memory of God and the memory of others can undoubtedly be dissonant and pastorally difficult. But that does not make the suggestion untrue. The fact that God will remember is the key to faithful hoping and Christ-like healing practice.

Memory without Neurology

It is a fact that God's memory is quite different from the type of memory we have been looking at in this exploration of human memory, if for no other reason than that God does not have a brain—at least in our sense of the word. As Dallas Willard once put it, "For God, everything is a no-brainer!"[294] This is serious point. When we use the term "memory" in relation to God, it is tempting to assume that God's memory is similar to human memory. When God remembers, we might think, he draws on his remarkable skills of recall and plumbs the depths of history for facts that have been stored in the divine database: *the book of life*. If God's memory is similar to human memory, only more comprehensive and more powerful, and if the reflections on human memory that have been presented are accurate, then being remembered by God is not particularly a comforting or stable prospect for any of us, demented or otherwise. If, like humans, God unintentionally forgets more about us than he remembers, and if God has no real idea of who we are, then divine memorial hope is at best fragile and at worst hopeless.

God's memory differs from human memory because it is not neurological, but also because his memory holds and remember us as we actually are, not simply as we think we are or have been. God searches us and knows us; thus, his memory will be full of surprises—some good and some not.

The suggestion that God remembers differently and that he does not have a neurological brain are not after thoughts. Like Augustine, many of us are used to the assumption that memory is something that emerges from and is confined within the biological brain. That God does not have such a brain but still remembers, clearly means the concept of memory is broader than our standard neurological and psychological definition, and memory may well not reside purely and simply within individual brains. Our standard accounts of memory reflect one aspect of what the term "memory" might mean. Divine memory opens up a whole new story around the nature of memory. God's memory is the place where all other memories are held.

Divine Memory as Sustenance and Action

Unlike human memory, God's memory does not simply recall events and actions, not least because past, present, and future are not concepts that can be applied to him. God sits outside of time, and thus there is, in a sense, no past to recall and no future to move forward. What God forgets ceases to exist; conversely, to be remembered is to be the recipient of divine action. Brevard Childs, in his book *Memory and Tradition in Israel*, offers extensive study on the Hebrew word for memory: *zkr*.

> God remembers and forgets, and this process stands parallel to a series of psychological descriptions (Jer. 31:20; 44:21). Of course, God's remembering has not only a psychological effect but an ontological one as well. Whoever Yahweh does not remember has no existence (Ps. 88:6). When God forgets sin, he forgives (Jer. 31:34).[295]

When God forgets something, it literally no longer exists. To be remembered is to exist and to be sustained by God. There is a close connection between memory and *nephesh*. To be forgotten is to have one's *nephesh* withdrawn; to cease to exist, to no longer be sustained by God. This explains why when God forgives sin, he forgets it in every sense—it literally no longer exists (Isa. 43:25). Redemption and the cleansing of human sin are literal events that occur within the memory of God.

As well as having a deep connection with sustenance, memory is deeply tied to action. Child observes that for the Hebrews, a human being was a whole person. The precise nature of that wholeness is important for an understanding of the nature of divine memory. For Hebrews, thought and illness were not merely contemplative aspects of persons. They were attitudes or inclinations toward particular forms of action. Contemplative perceptions of memory apart from action was unknown to the Hebrews. When the soul thinks, it acts.

Therefore, memory and action are seen to be thoroughly interconnected. Clearly, the emphasis is on remembrance-as-action directed toward someone.[296] When people remember, it is to enable action. The crucial parallel is this: *When God remembers, God acts.* God's memory is for the purpose of remembering. To remember something is to bring back together that which has been fragmented to one of wholeness in God: *Shalom.*

To be held and remembered by God implies some form of divine action toward the object of memory. It is something that occurs in the past and in the present as well as in the future. God acts in a particular way toward people because of a previous commitment—God remembers because God promises.[297] Most of all, God remembers his covenants, which existed before the creation (Gen. 1:26-28). God's remembering of his various covenants is not simply reflected in past history. The acts of any given covenant continue to meet Israel in the present and the future (Ps. 111:5). This is why the writer to the Hebrews can say with confidence that "Jesus Christ is the same yesterday and today and forever" (Heb. 13:8) and Jesus can proclaim, "I will be with you always, to the very end of the age" (Matt. 28:20).

Human memory is nothing more or less than one mode of participation in the memory of God, which is our true memory and our only real source of identity and hope. It becomes clear that to suggest that God remembers persons with advanced dementia is not a palliative avoidance of the real truth that they have lost their identity. Neither is it an abandonment of these people by God in the present. Quite contrary to that, it is a firm statement that God is *acting* with and for them and that God is acting with and for them in the present as they move toward his future with and for them.

Memory, Soul, and Resurrection

All of this is to get us to a clear understanding of what human identity might look like and how it might be sustained even in the most severe dementia. We are who we are because God remembers us and holds us in who we are. We are who we are now, and who we will be in the future will be because God will continue to remember us. Theologically, our identity relates to the person whom God sees and remembers This is a direct bearing not only on a person's endurance after their death and their identity when they have dementia, but on every moment that they exist.

To be remembered by God is to endure in the present and into eternity. This type of remembering, however, is not a matter of looking back and holding on to what was. For God, there is no "back" to look at, no "forward" to look toward. God is beyond time; for him, all is now. The important thing to bear in mind is that the movement from life to death is a movement from time into eternity, an eternity wherein our true identity is preserved in the memory of God. It is in this sense that we endure eternally.

That being so, while human beings forget many things, nothing is forgotten by God unless he chooses to forget.[298] Because there is no reason to think that God chose to forget those who have advanced dementia, there is no reason to suggest that a person's identity has been lost after encountering advanced dementia.

Our identity is safe in the memory of God. If God forgets us, we will cease to exist, but he does not forget us. As indicated previously, God's memory is not bound by time, space, or neurology in the way that "being remembered by God" is a prospective idea that finds fulfillment only in the future. Similarly, the present is equally misleading. Human memory may be fallible, constructed, and uncertain, but God's memory is sure and oriented toward action in the present.

Where Are Our Memories?

If memory requires action, then what kind of action does God's remembering bring about? It is all well and good to talk about God remembering us in the present and in the future, but if that is to be more than a mere platitude, we need to think through what such an assertion might look like when it is embodied. If God's memory necessarily includes action, where is that action to come from? What does it look like? Taking another look at Lisa Genova's novel *Still Alice* may help answer these questions.[299]

This novel tells the story of a fifty-year-old woman's sudden descent into early onset Alzheimer's disease. Alice's struggles to hold on to her sense self and to cope with her fast-disappearing past is an excellent narrative about the experience of the journey into dementia, Although fictional, it is deeply emphatic and authentic. One thing that keeps Alice going in the midst of her troubles is her Blackberry. It is the place where her appointments are kept, her cooking times are remembered and her life is organized. The various alarms that go off on her Blackberry alert her to do this or that, and she is able to negotiate the ever-increasing confusion of her life. Her Blackberry becomes her life. Alice has a secret stash of pills that she plans to use to end her life when she feels that she can no longer cope with her existence—when the Blackberry and other aids no longer make a difference. Not surprisingly, a powerful turning point occurs in the book when Alice loses her Blackberry. Eventually, it turns up in the freezer—but the frozen circuits in her telephone mark the end of its function as her memory. Alice later finds the pills she had hidden away and flushes them down the toilet. At this point, she cannot remember what they were for.

This story reveals something important—our memories are not simply in our heads or in our brains; they are scattered in many places. Our reflections on the nature of the memory of God indicate that our memories and our identity are not confined to the boundaries of our skulls; memory in a real sense clearly exists both inside and outside of individual brains. The memory of God, of course, is in the place where such memories exist and are sustained. But they exist in other places as well—places that we hardly notice or simply take for granted. For Alice, her telephone really was a critical part of her memory. It was not a substitute or compromise; it was truly part of her memory. Every time we take notes at a lecture or write down a shopping list, we are grafting in external aspects of our memory. Even within our constructions of our identities, it is often the memory of others that helps us to have memories of ourselves.

Memory is thus seen to be both internal and external. Some of it is held by the individual; some of is held by community or technology; all of it is held by God. Even in normal times, some of our memories are outside of ourselves and often stored and told by others around us. And when some things about ourselves are far from clear in our own minds, we are able to experience a sense of self through the memories of us held by those around us, through the stories they tell about us. Memory, like mind and personhood, is corporate through and through.

Remembering God; Remembered by Others

If our identity is held in and by the memory of God, then we can be certain that dementia does not destroy us now or in the future. That is the promise and the basis for enduring hope. But if being remembered by

God indicates and indeed necessitate some form of action in the present as well as in the future, then presumably God is doing something *right now* in the lives of people with severe dementia. That *something right now* has two dimensions, one of which, as we have seen, relates to the work of the Holy Spirit, as God is with the person who has dementia in ways that we cannot know. This dimension can be grasped only by faith. We trust that God is with and for the person even if we have no real idea of what that might mean. The Apostle Paul tells us,

> the Holy Spirit helps us in our weakness. For example . . .
> the Father who knows all hearts knows what the Spirit is
> saying, for the Spirit pleads for us believers in harmony
> with God's own will. (Rom. 8:26–7)

When we don't know what to say, the Spirit prays on our behalf. When we can no longer say what we want to say, the Holy Spirit intervenes on our behalf. When we can no longer access God through our prayers, our meditations or the Scriptures, we can be certain that God is with us in ways which, at least right now, we don't understand. In this sense, if and when we reach the advanced stages of dementia, we can be "sure of what we hope for and certain of what we do not see," as the writer to the Hebrews so poetically puts it (Heb. 11:1).

The second dimension is more observable and can be seen quite clearly through our communities. If people act toward us in ways that remind us that we are remembered, then we can see, feel, and touch God's memories in action. As we encounter others, we encounter God. If, as has been suggested, each encounter between human beings is an encounter with the Holy, then one vital dimension of God's active memory relates to the ways in which God's people encounter one another. It **is** as we remember the holiness of the person with dementia that we are able to act in sanctified ways. It is as we learn to meet people soul-to-soul—*nephesh*-to-*nephesh*—that the practice of remembering finds flesh and potency.

Soul to Soul: A Community Attention

When the church, as a living body of remembering others, learns what it means to hold onto and practice the right memories of healing and hope, then active remembrance becomes a practical possibility. It is true that the church is not the only community that needs to learn to remember well. Malicious social memory is present throughout society. The church, however, is the only community that exists solely to bear active witness to the living memory of Jesus. As such, it should be the place where people learn to see what God's memory looks like. These two dimensions—the work of Spirit and the faithful embodiment of God's Spirit (*nephesh*)—provide a hopeful practical theological basis for effective dementia care. Christians, therefore, are called to be attentive to the presence of God in others. If God is as close to human beings, then God is a God who experiences our sufferings and our joys. As we minister to one another, we minister to God; as we suffer in community, so God suffers with us. The church, then, is called to become an attentive community of memory and hope that understands what it means to remember people and to act accordingly. The memory of God creates a community of remembering that is called to learn what it means to be attentive to God in those for whom memory is no longer their defining feature or primary learning experience. Glen Weaver notes,

> Hebrew men and women experienced personal identity as they lived in community with other persons. God was revealed through historical events which established covenant with a people. The worship acceptable in God's sight was worship which emanated from the collective life of the people.[300]

It should be noted that identity is bestowed simply through the ongoing relationships of the community, as Kitwood affirms, but Weaver's point is deeper and safer for those with dementia. The community is the place where the implications of *nephesh*, which inspires and binds human beings together, are recognized and named and their Giver worshiped.

Such worship recognizes the obedience of humanity, the sovereignty of God, and the memory of God's great works. It is here, within the worshipping community, that our identity is sustained and upheld within both human and divine memory. As we realize that we are remembered, we are free to remember well. As we begin to forget, so others bear the weight of remembering for us, a form of remembrance that calls for quite specific forms of loving action.

The Memory of Resurrection

There is a point that needs to be clarified before we can see what such assistance to memory actions might look like. There is an important difference between the community of Hebrews and the community of the church—that difference is Jesus. For the Hebrews, God's *nephesh*, his breath of life, could be removed or withdrawn from an individual. When that happened, the person moved into death and was separated from God with no obvious way of reconciliation. Some of the angst that we encounter in the Psalms of lament relates to the recognition that a movement toward the extinction of a person's *nephesh* is a movement toward separation from God—that is, a complete loss of identity. Thus, things such as illness and suffering remind the Psalmist of death and separation from God and become a profound source of fear and existential angst. Psalm 88 ends with this plaintive cry:

> You have taken my companion and loved one from me;
> The darkness is my closet friend.

Whereas many of the other Psalms find resolution in the recognition of God's *nepheshed*—his unchanging love—Psalms 88 concludes with utter hopelessness. There is, of course, something important to be learned from this Psalm. Often, this is precisely how many people with dementia feel. Often, this is precisely how many people who care for people with dementia feel. It is alright to feel this way, even if staying in the pit may not be a good thing, but we need not remain in the depths. Jesus' resurrection has changed things, including the meaning of Psalms 88. It is certainly the case that the people may feel that the darkness is their closest friend. There is absolutely no doubt that the experience of dementia has a tendency to rip meaning, purpose, and hope from human lives. Darkness, however, need not be their final destination. In Jesus, we discover that we need not fear that God will withdraw his *nephesh*. It is certainly true that we will suffer and die, but neither experience is definitive of our stories. Reconciliation with God and in God has become a possibility for all people in all circumstances. Nothing can separate human beings from God's love—not death, loneliness, dementia, forgetfulness, anxiety, confusion, wordlessness—"nothing in all creation will ever be able to separate us from the love or God that is revealed in Christ Jesus our Lord" (Rom. 8:39).

The world has changed with the rising of Jesus Christ from the dead. That living, active memory provides a deep hope for all people, including those with dementia. Importantly, the resurrection is not an event that relates only to the past. In his words while initiating the Eucharist, Jesus said, "This is my body, which is given for you. Do this to remember me" (Luke 22:19). To remember Jesus is to bring him and the sacrifices and blessings that he represents into the present and to allow his memorial presence to change, challenge, and strengthen us. In the same vein, to remember Jesus' resurrection is not simply to look to the past or to the future, although it is timeless. It is also to look to the present and the significance of this great act of God as it works out its transforming power in the here and the now of human existence. This is an aspect of God's timelessness that takes on great significance for people with dementia:

> The upholding and renewing power of God is active in this present space and time. . . . Even the psalmists had an unclear anticipation of this truth when they confessed paradoxically that God was present even in the pit of darkness. But in another sense, this upholding, transforming power of the Spirit is the reality which now is the presence of the resurrected Christ—this body, the church. The church has the mission and the power to

renew creation. . . . In so doing, the church may bring to fulfillment the old testament vision that one's identity is established, redeemed, and maintained in the collective experience of a people living in covenant with their God.[301]

The memories of God are reflected and enacted in the memorial practices of the community that is gathered around the resurrected Christ. The power of resurrection is the binding force that underpins the community now and into the future. Even if our *nephesh* is moving upward toward its end or, as Weaver puts it, is returning to chaos, there are good reasons for hope in the present and for the future. It is precisely that hope that we engage within the Eucharist. God's active memory finds embodiment in the community of memory and resurrection. It is there, within that community, that we can discover what God's memory looks like.

Remembering people with dementia requires a community of attentiveness. To be attentive is to pay close attention to others. The church is called first of all to become a community that is attentive to God, the Rememberer and Bearer and Sustainer of our true identities. It is here that the church's worship finds its focus and goal. But the members of Christ's body are also called to become attentive to each other, and in particular to those among ones who may be considered weak and vulnerable (1 Cor. 12:21–31). A church that remembers well and is attentive to the needs of people with advanced dementia is a church that is remaining faithful.

11

Time Sense: Learning to Live in the Presence

"The friend of time doesn't spend all day saying: 'I haven't got time.'
He doesn't fight with time. He accepts it and cherishes it."

—Jean Vanier[302]

Jean Vanier, a French Canadian, a naval officer, and Aristotelian scholar, began a movement call "L'Arche"—which is French for "The Ark" in the biblical story of Noah and the Flood—the goal for which was to change the way that people with intellectual disabilities would be cared for. His intention was to invite them to come and share their lives in the spirit of the Gospel and the Beatitudes of Jesus.[303] Vanier wanted to live with them not as caregivers and care recipients but simply as friends. His initial pattern for community and relationships established the template for the beginning of a worldwide movement now known as the International Federation of L'Arche Communities. His interest was not in dementia, but it is an aspect of his theology and practice that holds particular relevance. At the heart of his perspective lies a rethinking of the nature, value, and use of time. He makes the following statement:

> Members of a community have to be friends of time. They
> have to learn that many things will resolve themselves if

they are given enough time. It can be a great mistake to want, in the name of clarity and truth, to push things too quickly to a resolution. Some people enjoy confrontation and highlighting divisions. This is not always healthy. *It is better to be a fiend of time.* But clearly too, people should not pretend that problems don't exist by refusing to listen to the rumbling of discontent; they must be aware of the tensions.[304]

Vanier's point is that in order to truly be with a person who has severe intellectual disabilities, it is necessary to re-orient one's sense of time. Within capitalist society, it is an almost irresistible temptation to treat time as one would treat any other commodity. Many of us spend much of our lives at war with time. Time rules us and dictates the nature and shape of our lives and relationships. Finding time to be with each other is not always a priority in lives where time seems to be racing away from us. Time is an extremely precious commodity. To be with someone with severe intellectual disability, we need to slow down and take time to notice those small things that the world sees as unimportant, but which, when we take time, are revealed to be profound. In *There is a bridge*, Stanley Hauerwas moves Vanier's ideas into the realm of dementia:

> To become a friend with someone with Alzheimer's, is exactly the kind of challenge that it means to become a friend of time. We forget that our most precious gift for others is presence; just being present. . . . Where there is not a lot to do other than to be present, you find out . . . what it means to be a friend of time.[305]

One profound way in which God remembers us is by being present with us.[306] A deep way of remembering a person with dementia is by being present with them. Memory and presence form the basis for the profound act of being with another without doing anything for them. This is the way Vanier has had to learn during his life with people who have severe intellectual disabilities. It is the same practice of presence for people as they encounter those who with advanced dementia.

The basic argument is this: *To love one another, one needs to be present for one another.* To be present, we need to learn to remember well and to use time differently and more faithfully. Then, we will discover that being with another is the most powerful way of ministering, not simply with and toward people with dementia, but also with and toward all people. As the community remembers and learns the rhythms of being with one another without the need for words, so healing can begin, even in the midst of deep forgetfulness. Then our task will be discovered and we will learn what it means to engage in such willful love.

The Knowing of Time

What is time and how is time and our perceptions of time shaped by our social context? Time is perceived as a pseudo-physical commodity to be bartered in the marketplace of temporal/spatial existence. It is valuable and can never get enough of it. Sometimes it becomes more of an enemy than a friend. Why does time have such a hold on us?

St. Augustine wrestles with the question: What God was doing before he created the world?

> Our God is the Creator of every creature in heaven and on earth. . . . If in term of Creator of "heaven and earth" he did not make anything at all. For if He did, what did He make unless it were creature. I do indeed wish that I knew all that I desire to know my profit as surely as I know that no creature was made before any creature was made.[307]

Augustine's concern is that if time existed before the creation of the world, this would involve the Creator in time. For him, the absolute contingency of the world is crucial. Time relates closely to non-being. If

God is in time, then God is open to this possibility, which reduces the contingency of creation.

> It is the tendency towards non-being that distinguished the temporal from the eternal because "should the present be always present, and should it not pass into time past, truly it could not be time but eternity."[308]

If God were subject to time, this would contradict the idea that God stands outside of time. It is wrong headed to ask that question. Time came into existence when the world was created; thus, time is an aspect of creation. Creaturely ideas about time should not be attributed to God.

> Therefore, since you are the maker of all times, if there was a time before you made heaven and earth, why do they say that you rested from work? You made that every time, and no times could pass by before you made those times. But if there was no time before heaven and earth, why do they ask what you did then? There was no "then," where there was no time.[309]

The implication of all of this is that time, as an aspect of creation, inevitably is fallen and in need of redemption. Thus, it is not really surprising that we have turned time into a commodity designed to enhance human wealth and productivity rather than taking time to bring glory to God the Creator or be with God's creatures. Such a perspective on time helps us understand more fully Paul's words in Ephesians 5:15–16: "See then that you walk circumspectly, not as fools but as wise, redeeming the time, because the days are evil" (NKJV).

Time and Care

Our culturally constructed assumptions about time impact the ways in which we choose to frame our practice of care. Time and caring are closely linked. Like the issue of "busyness," if we are not busy, then we probably are not working hard enough or caring effectively. It appears that we are not doing anything. To be busy doing things for people is to be working; to simply be with people is not. The problem is we tend to be so busy doing things for people that we cease to be with people in any meaningful way. Western culture, with its secular notion of time as acquiring meaning only through human plans and purposes, views unplanned time as empty time. If we see the time spent with people who have advanced dementia as empty time, then the experience of being present inevitably will appear meaningless and purposeless, and the significance of unique moments tragically will pass ones by.

The Keys to Our Memory

Jimmie was a former sailor whose memory was destroyed by Korsakov's syndrome. Arguably a specific form of dementia, this syndrome is the product of long-term alcohol abuse, which leads to irreversible degeneration of the brain. Jimmie's story is told in neurologist Oliver Sacks's book, *The Man Who Mistook His Wife for a Hat*. One of its central features is profound memory loss. The loss is so profound that most sufferers become people without any sense of a past or a future, trapped in an eternal present and bound permanently within one period of time. In a real sense, people with this form of dementia are lost and unable to establish roots. Strangely, Jimmie could remember things prior to 1945— but nothing since then.

Jimmie was easily able to forget a conversation, even after spending time talking at length with about his life and his memories prior to 1945. In a matter of seconds, his conversation with someone would have disappeared from his memory, and he would start his encounter with that person all over again. The disease had stripped him of something essential to what he was as a human being. From the neurological perspective, the person Jimmie had been was gone—his soul was gone. Such experiences with people who have neurological conditions that are odd, sometimes disturbing, are always deeply challenging and illuminating.

Those closest to Jimmie saw something different. Sacks was told by one of them to watch Jimmie in chapel:

> He did, and was profoundly moved and impressed, because he saw here an intensity and steadfastness of attention and concentration that he had never seen before in Jimmie or conceived him capable of.... Fully, intensely, quietude of absolute concentration and attention, partook of the Holy Communion, he was wholly held, absorbed by a feeling. There was no forgetting, no Korsakov's then, nor did it seem possible or imaginable that there should be.[310]

Something sacred happened to Jimmie when he entered the holy spaces of the chapel. Sack further observed:

> Clearly Jimmie found himself, found continuity and reality, in the absoluteness of spiritual attention and act. The one who pointed out this phenomenon about Jimmie is right, he did find his there. "A man does not consist of memory alone. He has feeling, will, sensibility, moral being.... It is here ... you may touch him, and see a profound change." Memory, mental activity, mind alone could not hold him; but moral attention and action could hold him completely.[311]

From Jimmie's perspective, his spiritual encounter allowed him to enter into a familiar narrative that provided him with an anchor and a sense of self that otherwise seemed to be missing from his life. The fact that he would have forgotten it soon afterwards is beside the point. The intensity and power of that unique and special moment was the transformative force that held him, made his life hopeful, and changed the perspectives of those who knew him from hopelessness to hopefulness. This change of perspective allowed others to hold Jimmie well. And this hope was stable. Jimmie responded in similar ways to certain other phenomena, but this was different:

> There was something that endured and survived. If Jimmie was briefly "held" by a task or puzzle or game or calculation, held in the purely mental challenge of these, he would fall apart as soon as they were done, into the abyss of his nothingness, his amnesia. But if he was held in emotional and spiritual attention—in the contemplation of nature or art, in listening to music, in taking part in the Mass in chapel—the attention, its "mood," its quietude, would persist for a while, and there would be in him a pensiveness and peace we rarely, if ever, saw during the rest of his life at the Home. I have known Jimmie now for nine years—and neurologically, he has not changed in the least. He still has the severest, most devastating Korsakov's, cannot remember isolated items for more than a few seconds, and has dense amnesia going back to 1945. But humanly, spiritually, he is at times a different man altogether—no longer fluttering, bored, and lost, but deeply attentive to the beauty and soul of the world.[312]

At one level, Jimmie's responses are understandable neurologically. The place in the brain that process art and music are close to the places where memories are stored, so the fact that such things might stimulate memory would seem to make some neurological sense. This is not, however, the only story that is worthy to tell because Jimmie's experience also makes theological sense. Think of it this way, when we listen to music, or at least when we are doing so in a more concentrated and intentional manner, we don't simply hum and sing along in a neutral way. Certain songs contain memories. As soon as we hear them, we are whisked backward in time to situations, events, and people that were deeply meaningful to us and that remind us of thing we have done and people we have loved. Such memories are laden with feelings and emotions. Music is a vehicle that we use as we travel through time.; it brings us back to often-forgotten destinations, some of which we remember with joy, others with sadness. Understood in this way, one can see that things such as song music, art, dance, and ritual actually function as modes of extended memory—that is, places where memory is stored external to its normal location in the brain. They act as keys that can unlock emotions, feelings, and recollections that otherwise would be inaccessible. People may be able to access certain memories via the normal processes, but whether it is music, art, prayer, or something else, they are keys that allow aspects of memory to be unlocked and accessed even if that access is only temporary and sporadic. When we watch someone with dementia move to the rhythm of music, when we see them dance without words, they may well be remembering cognitively or bodily something profound and deep about themselves and their pasts.

Likewise, when a person is caught up in a familiar prayer or hymn, or when they simply clap their hands to the rhythm of a song, they may well be remembering, cognitively or bodily, experiences they have had with God—or they may be having a new experience with God at that very moment. If we are to remember Jesus in the Eucharist, we must remember that remembering take many forms. Jimmie's increased functioning in the context of worship may well have had neurological explanations, but that does not mean what was happening was only neurological. The suggestion that Christian practices may act as keys to unlock memories takes us to a different place and allow us to tell different story and hold people like Jimmie quite differently. It enables us, like Michael Ignatieff's philosopher's son, to give him the benefit of the doubt. Jimmie's experience at Mass is similar to the presence of the students for Ann Goldingay and wordless Quaker worship for Mary; the acts of presence and worship became a vital place of reconnection with God and others. The experience of the wife of Jean Vanier's friends as she temporarily moved out of the fog is not incidental or meaningless. Even though the emergence may be fleeting, it is nonetheless real.

To be present with and for people with dementia is to fellowship and worship with them and to remember them well and to act accordingly. It is to hold them in their identities as people remembered by God and by the community of God's friends. We do people who suffer from dementia a huge disservice if we simply assume that their moments of springing to life are nothing but instances of meaningless procedural memory. If we fail to be with them in those moments—that will not be remembered and which may not return—we fail to remember them well and we will not act well toward them.

Be Friends with Time

To be in the moment with someone means that we have to change our conceptions of time. John Goldingay's "in the moment she will appreciate you," and Sack's words about Jimmie, "deeply attentive to the beauty and soul of the world," despite his profound memory loss—all draw our attention to the significance of time and the present moment. Humans as time travelers, through our use of memory, are constantly moving back and forth in time, reflecting on our past, thinking about the present, and looking forward to the future. Rarely do we slow down and take time to consider the meaning and significance of the present moment.

Ann for Goldingay and Jimmie for Sack had two uniquely different experiences of disability. Yet, at the heart of each was a common experience of the importance of the present moment. Jimmie's past eluded him, and because of that his future was unclear. Ann's disability meant that she could not articulate a sense of movement through history. The forward thrust of time as it took her from where she was to where she hoped to be going was elusive and evasive. Each experience involved a different mode of time, not spatial or progressive but at the same time deeply intentional and profoundly revealing. For both, "the now" held particular significance.

Becoming a friend of time is so vital and radical, as Vanier and Hauser suggest. Time provides existential space within which we learn to love and care for one another. But time needs to be sanctified, redeemed, and drawn into the service of God. We do this by simply slowing down and reclaiming time for its proper purpose. To learn to be in the present moment is to learn what it means to redeem time. We have all the time we need, we just need to learn how to use it faithfully. Hauserwas point out:

> Patience creates the time necessary for people to come
> to reconciliation and knowledge of one another in a way
> that we're not threatened to eliminate the other because
> that frightens us so deeply. We have all the time we need
> in a world that doesn't think it's got much time at all to
> draw on God's love, to enact that love, that the world
> might see what it means to be chosen by God.[313]

We are called to learn what it means to be in the moment, to notice the small things that the world rejects or explains away. We need to learn to live differently with time. To do so requires that we recognize where it is that we are living. If the world is actually creation, then we live in God's created time, and God created time for a purpose. Time does not just happen; it is created by God, sustained by God, and if we take time to listen, directed by God. Time matters. Living in God's created time means, if nothing else, that time is intentional, meaningful, and purposeful.

Calling by Name: Naming and Holding

The idea of being in the moment has wider implications and deeper meaning as it relates to the type of intimate experiences we have looked at so far. When we are the people in the moment, we learn what it means to name others properly and to hold them faithfully in that identity. To name something or label someone as having "dementia" has quite specific and typically negative connotations, socially, theologically, and neurologically. To slow down, take time, and gently call them by name is to hold them in their identity and make a strong statement about who we think they are and how we believe they should be treated.

It matters how we name things because naming determines what we see. In Exodus 3:4, God called Moses by name:

> When the Lord saw that he had gone over to look the burning bush, God called to him from within the bush, "Moses, Moses!" And Moses said, "Here I am."

In the sacrament of the present moment, we call out names of those whom we love and seek to offer care, and then we listen. But if we truly are with someone, we recognize and hear. To call someone's name is to give them the benefit of doubt. To listen for an answer is to show that we are willing to love. John Goldingay says this:

> As a human being, I am a person called by name—by God, and by another human being. In addressing disabled people by name, we affirm to them that they are and who they are. We affirm our love for them, and loving, but at least as much it expresses loving and thus facilitates knowing. Somehow this has implications to affirm our love for them, which operates despite or because neither we nor they may yet know much of who they are. Naming reflects knowing and loving, but at least as much it expresses loving and thus facilitates knowing. Somehow this has implications for people such as those with Alzheimer's disease who may be so profoundly mentally disabled that we may wonder what their "knowing" of themselves may mean. "They may no longer 'Know' who they are, but the church knows who they are." Oftentimes, it may be apparent that addressing them by name is received as an affirmation of love which meets with a response of love and trust. The one who names thus receives in return the gift of being loved and trusted and is built up.[314]

Naming something properly is an affirmation of worth and recognition and an important way of holding and remembering. To learn someone's name takes time.

The Sacrament of the Present Moment Soulful Companioning

To be with one another in the present moment is to allow our souls to touch. Meeting in the present moment is meeting soul to soul (*nephesh* to *nephesh*); it is a place where human souls encounter the soul of God. From this vantage point, we can understand why it is that for Ann and Jimmie, though perhaps in different ways, it was the present moment that formed their places of meeting with those who knew their names, remembered them, and held them in that sacramental place of remembrance. M. F. Eagan says, "A sacrament is, first of all, a sign of grace; that it is to say, it is an object or an action which, in virtue of some natural quality of its own, is capable of representing the supernatural and interior power of divine grace."[315] The presence of Ann 's friends, and their practice of slowing down and taking time with her was viewed as sacramental insofar as their actions and presence represents the reality of the presence of the Spirit of God as he remembers her and seeks to minister to her in and through the practice of the presence of God's people. God is in the moment, in the moment that God has created, and in the Spirit that brings into life and sustains two creatures as they encounter one another in this sacred time.

In the moment of Sack's revelation, it was only as he slowed down, and moved beyond those things that he had been trained to see, that he saw Jimmie in a close and intimate way and was able to see his soul. It was as he learned to remember Jimmie differently that love became a possibility for Jimmie's existence in the world. It should be noted that being in the moment is not necessarily a mystical experience or some kind of unearthly revelation given from on high. The sacrament of the present moment simply means providing the opportunities and having the epistemological awareness to allow people to notice things they never could have noticed before, and in noticing them, to see and respond differently. To be with someone in the moment is to be open to surprises, new possibilities, and these kinds of hidden experiences of people with dementia.

Learning to be in the moment is not necessarily a supernatural achievement, or what we usually refer to as supernatural. Thomas Merton once said, "the gate of heaven is everywhere."[316] There is real sense in which heaven and earth overlap within the earthiness of human beings. Jesus is not suggesting a picture of the world as some sort of Platonic reflection of an ideal version when he says, "Thy will be done on earth as in heaven." The gate of heaven is everywhere, wherein heaven and earth constantly overlap and intersect. This is also the case in and between human beings. The souls of people cannot be at peace with God, yet he is no **stranger** to our world. He is in every moment, but there are times when the present moment is all that there seems to be, and God's enduring attention in the present moment becomes a primary and ongoing place for revelation and worship.

There are more stories in Appendix F, "Hospitality among Strangers," that may help to sooth the feelings of those who involved with the dementia.

12

Natural Aging Versus Alzheimer's

Everyone knows that as we get older, our brain and body become weaker. In a natural aging process, it means that we may experience a slowdown in thinking and movement, *but our intelligence is not affected.* On the other hand, in the case of Alzheimer's disease, damage to nerve cells in the brain will cause *memory changes to worsen as more cells are damaged.* Although it is possible to develop Alzheimer's at any age, as young as 30, in most cases it affects parsons aged 65 and over.

Changes in memory caused by old age will be related to the names of people or places, but changes caused by Alzheimer's are expressed through forgetfulness that severely affects one's ability to work and even engage in a social life and hobbies. It is recommended to become familiar with the following ten warning signs to help determine whether what you are experiencing is a natural aging process or the development of Alzheimer's disease. If you notice these signs in your parents or even in yourself, it is recommended to see your doctor to confirm or refute your concerns:

Memory loss that interferes with everyday life: Poor judgment and decision-making. One of the most common signs of Alzheimer's, especially in the early stages of the disease, is the forgetting of recently learned information. Other signs include forgetting important dates or events, repeating the same question again and again, relying heavily on memory aids (e.g., notes) or family members for things that one normally would be able to take care of themselves until recently. **Age-Related Changes:** Making a bad decision occasionally. If sometimes you or your parents forget or miss a meeting, but remember it after some time, it is a sign that it is just old age and not Alzheimer's. If the memory problem does not interfere with normal functioning and does not makes you forget many things and feel confused, you do not have to worry too much.

Difficulty in planning ahead or solving problems: Decreased planning ability to perform a task. Some people with Alzheimer's sometimes feels a change in their ability to plan and follow clear instructions, especially when working with numbers. For example, they find it difficult to cook using recipes or to keep track of monthly bills. In addition, many also suffer from concentration difficulties and take a long time to do things that they previously performed in a shorter time. **Age-Related Changes:** Lack of ability to focus. If you or your parents make mistakes in calculating your bills from time to time, this is not a sign of Alzheimer's disease but simply a lack of attention from the aging process. This is natural, and if you go over the numbers again, you probably will notice your mistakes.

Difficulty completing tasks at home, at work, or at leisure: Inability to manage a daily task. People with Alzheimer's often have difficulty completing simple daily tasks. They may have difficulty traveling to a place they have traveled to dozens of times before, working with numbers or even keeping track of the rules of a favorite game. **Age-Related Changes:** Missing payment due dates. If you or your parents occasionally need help getting the TV to work, or fixing a computer, or with constantly changing technology, which is hard even for a person without Alzheimer's, these are normal challenges that come with age.

Confusion about times and places: Losing track of the date or the season. People with Alzheimer's can completely forget today's date, what day it was yesterday, and even what season of the year they are in. In addition, they may have difficulty understanding processes that are not taking place immediately and sometimes even forget where they are going, where they are, and how they got there. **Age-Related Changes**: Forgetting which day it is and remembering it later. If you or your parents forget which day of the week it is, but then remember at some point, it is a sign of old age and not Alzheimer's. Keep in mind that sometimes even young people forget the day and date, and the reasons sometimes include a lack of weekly routine. This may be caused, for example, by retirement and losing the sense of the weekend compared to the rest of the week.

Difficulties in vision and understanding of images and spatial relations: Weaker eyesight. For some people, vision problems are a sign of Alzheimer's. These people will have difficulty reading, measuring distances, or noticing the differences between certain shades or colors. In addition, they may suffer from problems in spatial perception, such as not recognizing themselves when they pass a mirror, leading to them thinking someone is in the room with them. **Age-Related Changes:** More eye related disease. It is known that vision is impaired by aging and therefore blurred vision is not necessarily an early sign of Alzheimer's disease. In addition, a problem with vision can be related to other diseases, such as cataracts or diabetes, so once you notice these changes, you should consult your doctor to rule out the variety of possible problems.

Development of difficulties in using words orally and in writing: Difficulty recalling words. Difficulty having a conversation, losing their train of thought while talking, and repeating themselves several times without noticing. They can also have trouble using rich vocabulary or even finding the right name for objects and people that are familiar to them. This includes calling their children or their friends by incorrect names. **Age-Related Changes:** Sometimes forgetting which word to use. If you or your parents find it difficult to find the right word for what you want to say, it does not necessarily indicate the development of Alzheimer's disease. Aging causes many brain processes to slow down, and memory itself no longer functions as it did in the past. If you do not confuse words and call things by a name that does not belong to them, such a memory problem is not necessarily a sign of Alzheimer's disease.

Misplacing things and inability to retrace steps: Inability to retrace and find the missing thing. A person with Alzheimer's can place objects in places they do not belong without noticing, and often lose objects and fail to retrace the steps they took to help them find them. Sometimes Alzheimer's patients may even blame another person for stealing, and as the years go by and the disease worsens, this may occur more frequently. **Age-Related Changes:** Losing things from time to time. If you or your parents find it difficult to remember from time to time where you have put your glasses or the remote control, it is not necessarily a sign of Alzheimer's disease. It is possible that these are problems that you already have dealt with in the past but which are exacerbated by old age. If this is not an unreasonable case, such as leaving your shoes in the refrigerator, there is no reason to worry much.

Poor judgment and difficulty in making decisions: Inability to make sound judgments. For example, they may make poor decisions about money, being quick to hand out large amounts of money to telemarketers. In addition, they may pay less attention to cleanliness and grooming. **Age-Related Changes:** Easily falling into a scam. Making wrong decisions from time to time does not necessarily mean you have Alzheimer's disease. Telemarketers often are professionals who know how to "milk money" by using emotions rather than turning to logic. So even in this case, if you or your parents can still say "no thanks" and know that you do not need the product being sold, you have no reason for concern.

Avoiding social activities or work: Having the perception of falling behind updated knowledge. People with Alzheimer's may stop engaging in past hobbies and avoid social gatherings and/or anything related to work. They may even stop loving to watch football because they no longer are able to follow their favorite team. The reason for these changes is the perception of all the difficulties that accompany them, which makes them realize that something is wrong with them and that they cannot function as they did in the past. **Age-Related Changes:** If you or your parents feel exhausted from work or want to avoid social interaction, it is not necessarily a sign that Alzheimer's disease is involved. Exhaustion at an older age from work you have done over many years makes sense, and avoiding contact with friends, especially when you feel obligated, is only a sign that your body and mind need more rest than when you were younger.

Changes in mood and personality: These are not the same person any more People with Alzheimer's may become completely different people and respond to situations differently than they normally would. They may be confused, suspicious, depressed, anxious, or stressed. It may also be easy for them to succumb to sadness in the home and work environment, or experience depression while they are outside their comfort zone.

Age-Related Changes: Difficulty adapting to new settings. If you or your parents feel nervous or insecure after a change that someone or something creates in doing things and you are not ready to change them at this point in your life, that is not abnormal. Changes in routine at an older age would irritate and disturb anyone, so it is not necessarily a sign of Alzheimer's disease. Note that mood swings can also be signs of other illnesses, so you may want to check with your general practitioner.

Distinguishing between natural aging processes and Alzheimer's sometimes may be difficult. Keep in mind, however, that just because an older adult is forgetful does not mean that he or she has Alzheimer's disease. In fact, the cause of the problem might be side effects of medications, the most common form of reversible dementia. But if you or your parents experience some of the symptoms that are not age-related changes, you should consult your doctor for proper testing and treatment. It is also important to note that any such radical change alone may indicate other diseases, and therefore it is recommended not to rush to think that you might have Alzheimer's; rather, you should consult a doctor for a professional opinion.

Is It Dementia or Alzheimer's? Why Does It Matter?

The terms dementia and Alzheimer's have been around for more than a century, which means people likely have been mixing them up for that long. Knowing the difference is important. While Alzheimer's disease is the most common form of dementia, there are several other types (see Appendix D). The second most common form is vascular dementia, which has a much different cause—namely high-blood pressure. In addition to these two, there are other less common types of dementia, each of which has different causes as well. In addition, certain medical conditions can cause serious memory problems that resemble dementia.

A correct diagnosis means the right medicine, remedy, and support. For example, knowing that you have Alzheimer's instead of another type of dementia might lead to a prescription or cognition-enhancing drug instead of an antidepressant. Finally, you may be eligible to participate in a clinical trial for Alzheimer's if you have been specifically diagnosed with the disease.

What it is Dementia? Simply, it is a nonreversible decline in mental function. Several disorders can cause chronic-memory loss, personality changes, or impaired reasoning, with Alzheimer's disease being just one of them. To be diagnosed with dementia, the disorder must be severe enough to interfere with your daily life. On the other hand, Alzheimer's disease takes away the ability to carry out even the simplest tasks. There is no cure for Alzheimer's disease. Researchers have identified biological evidence of the disease—amyloidal plagues and tangles in the brain that can be seen microscopically, or more recently using Pet scan that employs a newly discovered tracer that binds to the proteins. You can also detect the presence of these proteins in cerebral spinal fluid, but that method is not often used in the U.S.

To diagnose dementia, a doctor must find that you have two or three cognitive areas in decline, such as disorientation, disorganization, language impairment, or memory loss. To make the diagnosis, a doctor or neurologist typically administers several mental-skill challenges. In the Hopkins verbal learning test, you try to memorize then recall a list of twelve words—and a few similar words may be thrown in to challenge you. Another test, also used to evaluate driving skills, involves drawing lines to connect a series of numbers and letters in a complicated sequence. In Alzheimer's, there is no definitive test; doctors mostly rely on observation and ruling out other possibilities. For decades, diagnosing

Alzheimer's disease has been a guessing game based on looking at a person's symptoms. A firm diagnosis was not possible until an autopsy was performed. The guessing game that is still used today has an accuracy rate of between 85–90%. The new PET scan has a 95% accuracy rate, but it is recommended only as a way to identify Alzheimer's in patients who have atypical symptoms.

Symptoms at Various Stages of Alzheimer's Disease

Have you noticed memory problems piling up in ways that affect daily life in yourself or someone you love? Do you find yourself struggling to follow a conversation or find the right word, becoming confused in new places, or botching tasks that once came easily? According to the Alzheimer's Association, more than five million American have Alzheimer's disease, and estimates suggest it will affect 11–16 million Americans by 2050. Already, it is the sixth leading cause of death in the U.S., according to a special Health Report on Alzheimer's Disease titled, "A Guide to Coping, Treatment, and Caregiving," which includes in-depth information on diagnosing Alzheimer's and treating its symptoms.

To help identify problems early, the Alzheimer's Association also created a list of ten warning signs for Alzheimer's disease that individuals may experience one or more of in different degrees[317] (which are similar to the specific signs listed above). There are also various similar lists by many other organizations.

Symptoms of Alzheimer's disease may progress through three stages:[318]

1. **Early stage**—people begin experiencing short-term memory deficits, difficulty in decision-making, problem in performing routine tasks, personality change and mood changes. The symptoms generally present themselves over a two-to four-year period.

2. **Middle Stage**—memory loss often worsens, communication skills weaken, reasoning becomes difficult, and attention to

personal care needs may diminish. The stage can last from two-to- ten years or more.

3. **Late Stage**—there is a further decrease in mental function and communication skills. People lose the ability to recognize family members and friends, they cease to speak and eat, lose muscle control and swallow reflexes, slip into coma, and eventually die. This stage lasts from a few months to three years. Keep in mind, there is no two persons experience the disease in the same way or at the same rate of progression.

However, Reisberg describes Alzheimer's disease progress in seven distinct clinical stages:[319]

1. **Normal stage**—no symptoms.
2. **Age-Associated Memory Impairment stage**—normal with symptoms. The person forgets where they have placed familiar objects or forgets names of people that were known previously. There are no other significant problems with memory.
3. **Mild Memory Impairment stage**—not normal, although not necessarily Alzheimer's disease. The person gets lost when traveling to unfamiliar locations, and their work performance declines. They have difficulty finding words, retain little when reading, and have concentration problems through memory testing. People at this stage still have enough awareness and insight to direct their personal business. This stage lasts about seven years.
4. **Mild Alzheimer's stage**—demonstrates decreased knowledge of current events; some loss of memory for important events in their life; and decreased ability to handle slightly complex tasks. The person does not have problems with orientation, recognizing familiar persons and faces. This stage lasts about two years.
5. **Moderate Alzheimer's stage**—Inability to recall major events of the person's current life or remembering names of familiar people and places. At this stage, they do not require assistance with daily

functions, and are not ready to be moved into care facilities. This stage lasts about one to two years.

6. **Moderately Severe Alzheimer's stage**—The person forgets their spouse's name occasionally and is largely unaware of events in their life. Usually they remain orientated to their surroundings. They may become incontinent, and personality, emotional, and delusional behaviors may change. Caregivers become unable to handle the person. This is the time nursing home placement occurs. This stage lasts about two to three years.

7. **Severe Alzheimer's stage**—The person's ability to move about, communicate, and understand are all lost as well as all basic self-care activities. Nursing home becomes inevitable because of heavy care demands. This stage lasts about two years, and some die shortly after onset of this stage; others may live much longer. The time from onset of the disease to death is approximately seven to eleven years or may be from two to fifteen years.

As has been stated, there is no treatment that can reverse or cure the effects of this mental disease. In research over recent years, however, several promising medications have been developed to slow down the disease process if prescribed early, which also may help to control symptoms and delay the progression of the illness.

13

Preventing, Slowing, and Prolonging Alzheimer's Disease

How can families avoid the dreaded condition altogether? Does science offer any hope? Will there be a cure, or are there preventive precautions to the much-feared Alzheimer's disease? The latest research confirms that proactive brain health (body as well) maintenance before and during the early stages of Alzheimer's and other dementias may slow the process of deterioration. Besides genetics, there are many other causes that may trigger dementia, including Alzheimer's: High blood pressure, weight gain, obesity, poor diet, depression, diabetes, lack of physical or mental exercises, smoking, excessive alcohol use, and lack of social or spiritual life. Positive responses to any of these factors will suggest a poor brain lifestyle that may contribute to dementia later in life. Since our brain is a part of our body, dementia is not just a concern for seniors but for everyone, young and old.

What about family members who want to help their senior loved ones and themselves avoid the dreaded condition altogether? Proactive brain health (healthy body and brain) maintenance before and during early stages of Alzheimer's may slow and slow the process of deterioration. Richard Powers, a neuropathologist and geriatric psychiatrist as well as a member of the Alzheimer's Foundation Board, shares that there is a great deal of misinformation about the cure and treatment of Alzheimer's and other dementias. In his *Handbook for Spiritual Communities on Helping*

Members with Memory Problem, he alerts the boomer generation on ten ways that recognizing dementia may help seniors:[320]

1. Correct treatable causes of memory trouble.
2. Slow the progress of some dementia.
3. Improve medical and hospital care.
4. Reduce risk for accidental injuries.
5. Avoid complications from over-the-counter medication.
6. Allow the parent to organize and safely manage their personal business.
7. Reduce risk of avoidable problems that cause a parent to move from their home.
8. Protect against financial exploitation.
9. Protect against abuse by others.
10. Improve the quality of everyone's life by reducing anxiety and stress.

Informed adults can make healthy lifestyle changes that decrease their risk of developing dementia. In the presence of a diagnosis, simple lifestyle modifications can lessen the unpleasant impact of dementia on both seniors and those who care for them.

Facilitate Spiritual Growth in Later Life

Most people—religious or secular—believe that facilitating spiritual growth ultimately is the most effective way of maintaining mental health, physical health, and vigor. We all know the mind has an enormous influence on the body, and the spirit has an enormous influence on the mind. Consequently, spiritual growth may even contribute to maintenance of physical health as people age.

Regardless who one is, because of the influence of spirituality over the mind and body, there are many reasons to pursue spiritual goals that go way beyond health. In fact, even if some spiritual goals were bad for health, they would be still be worth pursuing because, particular for people of faith, spiritual development and growth are to be sought after as ends in themselves, Indeed, while life and health here on earth are temporary for all of us, spiritual matters represent things of eternal, immeasurable value that need to eclipse all other priorities.

The aging process itself has a way of facilitating spiritual growth that clergy, religious caregivers, and even elderly persons themselves, would be hard pressed to compete with. Even in cases when people become angry at God and turn away from him because of stressful or traumatic life experiences, such as Alzheimer's disease or PTSD, and so on, loss, pain, and suffering are the surest goads to spiritual growth. Pastoral caregivers have an opportunity to straightforwardly address issues of faith with sufferers. C.S. Lewis said it well when he wrote, "Pain is God's megaphone to a deaf world." In religious work, it has found that those who become angry at God, or turn away from spiritual matters when bad things happen often did not have a truly meaningful relationship with God prior to these events. Seeing such traumatic, stressful events positively may be the catalyst leading to a new, deeper, and more intimate relationship with God, one that causes people to run toward, not away from God for comfort when tragedy strikes. As God is active in our spiritual growth, even when we suffer losses and traumatic experiences, clergy and religious caregivers can partner with God to facilitate the process of spiritual growth in later life. Following are four ways this can happen:

First, clergy can address the meaning and purpose of pain and loss in their sermons and crafts these homilies to meet the emotional needs of physically ill and/or aging persons in any worship service or congregation. Even younger adults need to understand the meaning of loss, tragedy, pain, suffering, dependency, and altruism; these topics are applicable to persons of all ages, for pain and love are experienced by young and old alike. Such topics will also make the content of sermons relevant to the daily lives of those in the caring facilities or churches.

Second, the focus of church services and church school needs to be directed toward the role of faith in coping with the everyday struggles of life. Indeed, God wants to be involved in our sufferings, failures, and triumph, in every aspect of our lives, regardless of age. Sermons and lessons that bring God into the daily lives of people as they struggle through their week will foster spiritual growth and bring persons closer to God. Even church potlucks and bazaars might be more directed to meet the needs of those less fortunate in the congregation or community, again sending the message that fostering spiritual growth and Christlike lives are the primary mission of the church. Spiritual growth, like any type of growth, is not always pleasant or comfortable.

Third, when counseling older adults who are going through life crises, clergy and religious caregivers should bring God into the situation as part of the solution. Relying on psychological principles and theories to understand and work through problems, while helpful, cannot replace the power of spiritual healing. If elders cannot draw on the strengths and comforts of their faith in God to help them work through their problems, then the counselor must thoroughly and carefully explore the person's religious history trying to identify previous negative experiences with religion or current misperceptions about God. These previous experiences may block the person's ability to receive comfort from God in the present situation and, once identified, can be reexamined so as to be helpful working through their life situations. A person cannot be forced or bullied into reliance on faith and God; rather, the spiritual caregiver must offer a flexible, open, and established understanding for the person, meeting them where they are in their current state of mind. This will set the stage for further progress at the person's own pace, along their own unique spiritual journey, which will best facilitate leading them closer to God, closer to fellow human beings, and closer to God's purpose for their life.

Fourth, as has been repeatedly emphasized throughout this book, elders should be encouraged to use their gifts, talents, and wisdom to serve God by generously giving of their time and talents to meet the needs of others. As they do this, they begin to live out the great commandment of loving God and loving neighbor, the hallmark of the Christian life. Finally, elders should be encouraged to develop a routine of regular meditation, Bible study, and worship, both privately and with others. These religious behaviors, when performed sincerely and wholeheartedly, will nourish their souls, foster uplifting bonds of fellowship, and give spiritual strength to love and serve God as they have been called to do.[321]

Connection Between Dementia and Loneliness

Due to their social network shrinking as they get older and family members and friends die, loneliness is a central experience for many people with dementia. This also has to do with the ways in which malicious social psychology drive their friends away. That people with dementia are lonely and socially isolated is in no small point due to the arguments that have been presented on the effects of relationships on neurology.

A 2007 article in the *Archives of General Psychiatry* on the role of loneliness in the development of Alzheimer's indicated that people who are lonely are twice as likely to develop Alzheimer's disease.[322] Robert Wilson, a professor of neuropsychology at Rush University Medical Center, has this comment on the implications of the study: "There are two ideas that we should take away. Number one is it suggests that loneliness really is a risk factor, and secondly in trying to understand that association we need to look outside the typical neurology." He said that result ruled out the possibility that loneliness is a reaction of dementia. "It may be that loneliness may affect systems in the brain dealing with cognition and memory, making lonely people more vulnerable to effects of age-related decline in neural pathways," he suggested, "We need to be aware that loneliness doesn't just have an emotional impact but a physical impact," he said.[323]

Rebecca Wood, chief executive of Alzheimer's Research Trust, made this comment on the study:

> This is an impressive study. It follows a large group of people for a significant period of time and comes up with startling findings that back up earlier studies examining social interaction and Alzheimer's risk. What I find particularly interesting about this study is the fact that it is an individual perception of being lonely rather

than their actual degree of social isolation that seems to correlate most closely with their risk of dementia symptoms. However, it is interesting that the people who die during the study and had demonstrated symptoms of dementia did not have relatively more physical signs of Alzheimer's disease in the brain.[324]

During Janelle S. Taylor's fascinating anthropological reflection on her experiences with her demented mother, she noticed the regularity with which friends, family, and others asked her the same question: "Does she recognize you?"[325] Taylor was struck by the apparent significance that this question seems to have for other people. For her, the question of whether or not her mother recognized her was not particularly significant, but for others it seems to be vital. In her essay, following the thinking of the philosopher Paul Ricoeur,[326] she highlights a dialectic between three meanings of term "recognition"—recognition as identification (of things), recognition of self, and recognition by an "other."[327]

In the recognition of things, there is a correlation between what we see and what we are able to name. When we see a chair, for example, we recognizes it as a chair and act accordingly. At this level, recognition is simply something that we do while trying to make sense of the world locating ourselves within it. Recognition of ourself is the ability to know who we are, to use that knowledge to assess and negotiate the world, and to hold and sustain our identity and our sense of self-in-the-world. According to these aspects of recognition, "Does she recognize you?" is politics and appears relatively straightforward.

The third aspect of recognition makes things more complex. Recognition by another requires relationship and community and inevitably takes us into the realm of social and the political. While the first two modes of recognition are something that we do for ourself, the third movement of recognition is a social process. It is in this third dimension that Taylor realizes what she considers to be the real meaning of the question, "Does she recognize you?" and the potential problem for her mother when such a question is highlighted:

When Taylor was asked, "Does she recognize you?" her friends, in Riceour's terms, were giving voice to the first of the three distinct "moments" in the "course of recognition." The second question concerned her mother's ability, as a sovereign self, to actively draw intellectual distinction among the subjects and people around her. Consequently, Ricouer's third and final "moment" was when the subject was granted social and political recognition by others. The questions essentially concerned her mother's ability, as a sovereign self, to actively draw intellectual distinction among the objects and the people around her and whether or not she was granted social and political recognition by others.[328]

Taylor's deep concern points to the reality that, in asking the question, "Does she recognize you," people are not moving between the first two understandings of the term "recognition." Rather, they are actually exploring the third aspect; thus, "no" is Taylor's answer. Something will change in the way in which her mother is recognized within the social and political realms. Taylor implies that her answer actually will be a social marker, that her mother will shift from being perceived as a person to being perceived as a nonperson, or at least a lesser person whose social and political recognition is about to be withdrawn.

Tied in with this point and important to understand, is Taylor's noticing how almost all of her mother's friends had simply drifted away following her diagnosis and her subsequent journey into dementia:

> It appears that middle-class U.S. friendships are not generally expected to bear the weight of deep and diffuse obligations to care. More like pleasure crafts than life raft, they are not built to brave the really rough waters— and these are rough, corrosive, bitter waters indeed. Dementia seems to act as a very powerful solvent on many kinds of social ties.[329]

Taylor doubts that many friendships survive dementia's onset. What she says about the U.S. could just easily be said about the U.K. or the E.U. The ways in which demented people lose their social networks and friends, sometimes gradually and sometimes quickly, is striking. Gordon's experience is a good example of this process of "unfriending." After he went into care with his Alzheimer's, his social circle shrank from a once wide and engaged circle to primarily his wife, his daughters, and one or two individuals who chose to make time for him. The other friends made excuses of being busy or having other priorities for not visiting. They thought it would be a waste of time because they knew Gordon would forget them easily. Dementia is different from other terminal illness in that it is a hard condition to be around.

David Shenk reflects on the experience of former president Ronald Reagan who developed Alzheimer's in his later years. In his book *The Forgetting: Alzheimer's: Portrait of an Epidemic,* he points out implications for people living in U.S.:

> As expected, Reagan's descent had progressed steadily, his memory lapses become a rule rather than the exception and it was to a point that it drove him into further isolation. Partly out of simple courtesy to Reagan and partly due to their own personal discomfort, many of his friends stopped visiting when he started having trouble recognizing them.[330]

If someone who has been one of the most powerful men in the world has difficulties holding his network of friendships, then what hope is there for Gordon? There is no doubt that it can be difficult to be with a person you know but that person has forgotten who you are and indeed who they are. At times, it takes a leap of faith to remember them as the person that we knew, but no matter what, our friends remain our friends, do they not? The ease with which people with dementia can be unfriended raises a dark question: What is it that we actually love in those we claim to love?

Loneliness and God

The nationwide epidemic of isolation affects nearly one in five Americans 65 and older. Loneliness and social isolation have measurably negative health effects. Lifestyle interventions that simultaneously target multiple risk factors could protect cognitive function in older adults and increased risk for cognitive decline. Having active social relationships is one of them.

Developing and nurturing a relationship with God is one way that many persons cope with loneliness. At any time and at any place we can always talk to God, whether we are awake at midnight or in pain or in fear or in distress, we can talk to him about our feelings. Someone once said that humans were created with a hole in their hearts and there will always be emptiness (loneliness) if we try to fill it with other things, because only God can fill the hole. Putting God where he rightfully belongs in our lives may help to bring peace and wholeness to our heart.

In addition to the deep, abiding need that each of us has for God, our Creator has seen fit to make humans with inherent social needs. The Bible clearly says that God wants us to fill those needs through fellowship with others (Heb. 10:24–5). For this reason, those who are lonely and but healthy enough should be encouraged to involve themselves in the religious community. In this way, elders will have contact with others and will increase the likelihood for social relationships to combat loneliness. The need for God's people to reach out and invest in each other's lives, and to inspire members of the congregation to meet each other's social needs, including older members, should be strongly and clearly empathized in the faith community.

The consoling words and many promises of Scripture have the power to dispel loneliness. When prolonged, the experience of loneliness and isolation among older persons can cause dementia. So how can such people be helped to minimize this cause of dementia?

Working Longer Could Benefit Both Health and Finances

Waiting to retire until after age 65 and drawing social security benefits later can significantly boost income (if you wait until age 67, you can collect social security while working full time with no penalties). Working beyond 65 also could benefit mental stimulation and social engagement.

According to a *Washington Post* article, a record number of people 85 and older are still working. In 2016 Census Bureau figures, there are between 1,000 and 3, 000 U.S. truckers aged 85 or older.[331]

It is projected that millions of workers age 65 and up will be self-employed, a grow that will grow faster than any other age group over the next four years. There are an estimated 11 million low-income working adults who have less than $400 in savings—a benchmark for financial insecurity according to a U.S. Federal Reserve study conducted in 2017.[332] The following, which includes financial factors, are among the many reasons that senior citizens are working longer:

- Life expectancies are growing and people overall are in better health. People who live longer may have to work longer to support themselves.
- Education levels are rising. Studies show that college-educated people tend to work longer and retire late because professional jobs require less physical work.
- Lingering effects of the recession, financial assets lost value (Coronavirus Pandemic factor).
- Lower interest rates that reduced the yield on many saving instruments.
- People not having saving enough or misjudged how much money they might need.
- Fewer people receiving pensions when they retire.

Evidence from some studies links working past the traditional retirement age of 65 with better health and longevity, which can reduce the chances of dementia and heart attack. The motivations for working longer are many:

- Helps seniors avoid social isolation and keep them connected to their communities.
- Adds meaning to their lives; they can achieve goals they set for themselves.

- Allows them to use their knowledge and experience; they feel valued by their employers.
- Helps them to stay physically and mentally healthy.

Health experts say that staying mentally, socially, and physically active is good for health. Working longer enables many people to maintain these activities and relationships. According to a Harvard Health Letter, mental stimulation and problem-solving help to maintain cognitive skills. Social engagement is associated with fighting off chronic disease, and remaining physically active can lead to better health and sharper thinking skills.[333]

A further reason told in an article, "I Am Going to Work until God Tells Me Not to."[334] It says: The American workforce is graying. Baby boomers are staying on their jobs longer and finding new jobs after retirement in record numbers. The surge in older workers can be attributed to multiple factors, such as the disappearance of company pensions, the increasing age to collect full Social Security, and the average growing lifespan.

Such extensive changes in the workforce will continue to affect the economy for decades to come. The trillions of post-retirement dollars earned will circulate through cruise ship companies, restaurants, retailers, realtors, and all sectors of the marketplace. Less-affluent, still working seniors are likely to use fewer government social benefits, and older workers will provide both a steady stream of labor in tight markets, as well as competing with younger workers for jobs. Though many are happy to be still on the job, others are working because they have to. La Verne Gaither, a 40-year-old United Airlines flight attendant and a volunteer at a nonprofit belongs to the former group, and Janet Beebe, who runs a nonprofit Breast Cancer Survivors' Network, belongs to the latter. Both are cancer survivors. Gaither cannot envision herself retiring. For her, an active life of enjoyable work, helping others, travel, social activities, and freedom that a full-time income imparts is too good to give up. She said, "I am not that grandparent that wants to sit at home watching the grandchildren. I will work until God tells me not to. He is going to give me some kind of sign."[335]

Beebe, 70, loves her "from-the-heart work" as a paid chief executive officer of a nonprofit providing and coordinating services for poor cancer patients. She and her husband dreamed of calling it quits at 65 and going on an Alaskan cruise, but that dream melted away when he turned 58 and started showing signs of Parkinson's disease. He had to retire early and she had to put him in a care facility a few years later that cost her almost $6,000 a month. "I am working because I have to," Beebe said, "We are burning through our 402(K) and Social Security checks."

Regarding rising life expectancy, in 2000, about one in ten American aged 65 to 74 (4.1 million) were still working. Today, it is about one in four, which is expected to grow to one in three (14 million) in roughly six years (2027). In 2026, among those 75 and older, the workforce participants will double from one in ten to one in five. The life expectancy, which was 70.8 in 1970 now stands at 78.6. Health bills eventually come due, and they are more expensive than ever. If they have not saved for retirement and health bills, they must keep working. Fear of those expenses is pushing some boomers to stay on the job to keep company sponsored health insurance. Though they qualify for Medicare at 65, any monthly premiums for additional coverage slice away at fixed incomes, and Medicare, as an example, does not cover James Beebe's needs. Boomers still need to work to stay financially afloat.

In a 2016 poll by Boston University's Center for Retirement Research, about half of older workers said they needed extra income to maintain their lifestyles. Thirty years ago, about one in three needed it. It is hard to say how many must work just to keep some of life's basics in place. Poverty for older Americans is hard to pin down because of difficulty in tracking benefits such as payment from 401(k)s. But the range in senior poverty is probably between 9–14%. In 2014, Social Security retirement provided 90% or more of income for about 21% of couples older than 65, and for about 43% for singles. The age to collect a full amount of Social Security retirement is also rising, keeping many in the workforce longer.[336]

14

Who and What Can Help to Deal with Alzheimer's Disease?

"For God hath not give us the spirit of fear, but of power, and of love, and of a sound mind." (2 Timothy 1:7)

No one knows how to prevent Alzheimer's disease or how to cure it, but dementia causes profound changes in a person's functional abilities. Sustained loss of memory and impairment of other intellectual functions cause dysfunction in daily living. At least one of the following cognitive disturbances must also be present: 1) aphasia, vague, or empty speech, 2) apraxia, impaired ability to execute motor functioning, 3) agnosia, failure to recognize or identify objects, and 4) disturbance in executive function, failure to think abstractly, to plan, initiate, sequence, and monitor and stop complex behavior.[337] Because the assessment is complex with wide ramification both to diagnose and to provide the appropriate caregiving skills, this is an area the church community can provide referral sources to utilize the appropriate specialists and agencies within the community. Individual caregivers may have no way of knowing about these or how to coordinate but church members may have personal experience with them. While a primary caregiver such as a spouse is vital, early in the process secondary caregivers also are required, something that in aging congregations is already becoming a necessary or even central pastoral task.

There are also new drugs in development, such as "Aricept," the benefit of which may temporarily halt the progression of the disease, but the cost and severe side effects weight against its benefits. There are two practices—stay mentally and spiritual health—that may help to some extent (however, even this is uncertain).

Maintaining Mental Health

Although mental health is largely in people's minds, many mental disorders like Alzheimer's are widely thought to be determined by hereditary factors or biological diseases, which are not afflictions an aging person can control. In general, aging persons can best maintain their mental health by staying socially active and involved. It is strongly recommended as well to avoid alcohol and drugs to cope with life's problems, and choosing to think and behave in healthy ways that reduce psychological stress.

It has been normal in gerontology to associate aging with withdrawal from interaction with others and an increase in introversion. This become known as the disengagement theory of aging; in other words, it was thought to be a normal occurrence as people grew older. This theory proved to be incorrect, however, and was replaced by "activity theory" as a model for normal, healthy aging. This theory maintains that physical and mental activity that fosters involvement in social relationships increases the likelihood that people will age successfully.

Human beings are social creatures and require ongoing contact with others to remain mentally healthy, just as their bodies require nutrition to remain physically healthy. Equally important is avoidance of substances such as alcohol and drugs that adversely affect physiological changes to the body. Likewise, regular exercise and good sleep habits are important to stay physically and mentally healthy.

Especially during times of major life stressors, exercising positive thinking and cooperating with the Holy Spirit is beneficial to prevent many emotional problems. Timeless keys to mental health in late life are thought, belief, and behavior that stems from faith in God, which have been proclaimed for thousands of years as contributing to spiritual growth and maturation in the Judeo-Christian tradition. This is also the most powerful prescription for mental and spiritual health, which are so essential as persons age and lose their grasp on the things of the world that they once held with confidence. Science has demonstrated over and over that trust and faith in God provide mental stability during the aging process.[338]

Studies of older persons with chronical illness show that when their religious faith is strong, they recover more quickly than those who do not have this source of strength.[339] Especially if a person relies on the goodwill of others for their psychological strength to sustain emotional wellbeing, when others lose their ability to comfort, a relationship with God will become more and more important.

There is no guarantee of stability of good health or that good friends will be there forever. Principles of modern psychology often are not particularly useful in response to major life stressors. When physical disabling calamities strike and friends die or relocate, emotional support is diminished, but a person's faith is a constant source of comfort, especially when left alone with no one to depend on. Research indicates faith becomes the important source for wellbeing when stress is the highest and circumstance are the dimmest.[340] Religious faith can help people not to give up and have their emotional wellbeing built on a foundation of rock that will not fall even under such trying circumstances. This describes the one who has strong faith to sustain emotional wellbeing, while others' houses are built on sand; when the storms and heavy rains, they will be washed away (Matt. 7:26-7).

Centering your life on God and devoting your life to serving others in need will encounter many pitfalls and roadblocks that can dishearten even the strongest and most faithful individual, but the ultimate spiritual benefits will bring long-term mental health. The happiest older adults are those generous souls who give of themselves in service to others, abandoning their own self-centered preoccupations. One easy way to get involved is through volunteering, something that virtually all organizations are in need of and welcome wholeheartedly.

Maintaining Spiritual Health

Ultimately, this is the most effective way of maintaining mental health. The mind has an enormous influence on the body, and the spirit has an enormous influence on the mind. Therefore, spiritual growth may even contribute to the maintenance of physical health as we age. Regardless, there are reasons to pursue spiritual goals that go way beyond health. Spiritual development and growth are to be sought after as ends in themselves. It is touching things of eternal, immeasurable value that need to eclipse all other priorities. The aging process in later life has a way of facilitating spiritual growth one would be hard pressed to find a more effective substitute.

In a recent study at Duke Hospital of 87 elder patients who had multiple illnesses and were in great distress over their conditions, those who scored highest on intrinsic religiosity (or personal faith in God) recovered significantly faster from emotional distress than did persons with lower intrinsic religiosity.[341] In fact, having religious faith had an even greater effect on emotional healing than did changes to physical health and functioning. These results provide solid scientific evidence that intrinsically motivated faith (by placing trust and faith in God) helps older persons to better cope with chronic physical health problems. This was their most common response, that by simply turning their situations over to God and letting God take care of them (after doing what they could to solve their problems), they then were able to stop worrying and stop trying to work the situations out by themselves.

It is the preoccupation with and ruminating over a situation the person cannot change that generates negative emotions, so those with faith are able to release the worry back to God. Some of the elderly resolved to cope by praying that God somehow would bring them to comfort. Even though they had no control over the situation, they believed God did and that he would respond to their prayers and take care of things. This brought consolation and relief from worry or depression.

Reading the Bible and inspirational literature were other ways to cope by older persons that made them feel better. Singing religious hymns lifted the spirits of some. Visitation by clergy, or church members helped them to cope as well. Knowing that others have prayed for them during church services often has brought great comfort. Church attendance is always important to older persons, who often make extraordinary efforts to get to church despite functional limitations.

Clergy and religious caregivers have a great responsibility to help the older persons to use their faith to help them cope with illness. Here are some suggestions for these leaders:

1. Elders need to have a relationship with God and believe that he has their interests at heart. If human beings' existence is not simply a random or chance event in nature, then there must be some purpose and greater design for their continued presence here on earth. Spiritual leaders can help elders to realize and remember God's steadfast presence, that he always has their interests in heart, that he has a purpose for their lives, that he will give them a sense that they are not alone in their struggle, and that they are not in the hands of aimless fate. They need to be encouraged and taught to learn to stop struggling and to trust God to do what they cannot.

2. Unlike an older person's family, God always has their interests in heart. He has known them from birth, and understands everything that they are going through. Such reminders make elders feel less alone. Thus, encouraging them to talk with God about their fears and deepest concerns can help to counteract the isolation that accompanies the illness. Leaders can bring comfort and hope by reaffirming with the elderly that they are part of a Christian community (a praying group or praying chain) that commits to praying for them and their needs.

3. Sharing passages from the Bible with elders and encouraging them to think about and meditate on these passages will bring them comfort, especially the passages that are particularly applicable to their situation and. Biblical role models exist for almost every situation, especially those who are facing illness or tragedy in their lives. Explaining to them how these passages are

relevant to them can be comforting. Listening as they reflect on biblical truths, and allowing them to think aloud as they work through their own thoughts and feelings can be an invaluable gift to them.

4. Religious rituals (e.g., Confession for Catholics and Communion for most denominations) may be comforting and convey a sense of God's presence. Facilitating elders to attend church service and to participate in these rituals may be quite important to them in coping with their illness. Receiving Communion reminds them of Christ's suffering and death, and reaffirms God's deep love and commitment. Confessing sin may help prevent them from turning away from God in their present difficulties and instead to turn toward him. Other equally helpful and edifying actions: Encouraging them to use their faith in their circumstance; providing them with religious material and opportunities that may facilitate this; and allowing them to talk about and walk through their distrust of God, negative experiences with religion, or guilt over past sins. All of these actions can help the elder to access effectively utilize spiritual resources.[342]

Reflecting back to the story of Pete and Pam, how could church clergy and religious care-givers help, if they were members of their congregation? They may become angry at God and run away from him because of stressful or traumatic life experiences such as loss, pain, and suffering. What can clergy and religious caregivers do to work with God as partners to facilitate the process leading to a new or renewed relationship with God in later life? Following are five suggestions:

First, clergy can address in sermons the meaning and purpose of pain and loss, crafting these homilies to meet the emotional needs of those dealing with physical illness, suffering, dependency, and other crises that impact the daily lives of those in the church.

Second, church services and schools can focus on the need for faith in coping with every day struggles of life that brings God into their daily lives. Persons with strong religious faith have their emotional wellbeing built on a rock foundation that will not fall even under such trying circumstances as death or sudden disability.

Third, when counseling those older adults who are going through crises, clergy and religious caregivers should bring God into the situation as part of the solution. God wants to be involved in our suffering, failures, and triumphs, in every aspect of our lives, regardless of age. Relying on psychological principles and theories to understand and work through problems, while helping, cannot replace the power of spiritual healing. The elders can draw on the strengths and comforts of religious faith and faith in God in working through their problem. This will set the stage for future progress on their spiritual journey that will lead them closer to God, closer to their fellow human beings, and closer to God's purpose for their lives.

Fourth, elders should be encouraged to use their gifts, talents, and wisdom to serve God and to meet the needs of others. One of the best ways to maintain mental health as persons grow older is to invest energy and time into loving and serving God and the needs of others whose needs are greater. Being generous with one's time and resources provides a mindset that will bring fulfillment and mental stability to the aging person. Someone once said that you cannot find happiness, no matter how hard you try, you can only provide it to others and in doing so, you will experience it yourself.

Fifth, God uses people—human beings live in an action- and results-oriented society that does not value caregivers, or those who need such care or ministry. In our society, how can the life of someone who is severely dependent, demented, or even unconscious have meaning or purpose? Demented or uncommunicative persons may passively participate in God's love for the world by providing others with opportunity to provide love and care for them. An elderly grandparent who is in the nursing home with advanced Parkinson's disease may receive joy from watching her grandchildren become less self-centered and more focused on others as when they are visiting the grandparent. Alternatively, a severely disabled elderly person may see emotional and spiritual maturation in relatives who must put their own needs second to the disabled person's needs. Pastoral roles are to help both caregivers and elders recognize the mutuality of meaning, purpose, and joy in the reciprocity of caring and being cared for, and teaching them both the important role that human beings, regardless of their physical or mental state, can play in God's love for the world.

Fighting Back against Dementia and Alzheimer's

In the U.S., almost six million people are living with age-related dementias—about 70% of those cases are because of Alzheimer's disease. More than 89% of those folks are 75 or older, but 200,000 are younger than 65. In 2019 alone, 487,000 people over age 65 developed Alzheimer's disease. At the time of writing, it was estimated that one in every six women and one in every ten men living past age 55 would develop some form of dementia. Additional bad news is that medications to treat Alzheimer's disease essentially have missed the mark time after time. From 1999 to 2017, there were about 146 failed attempts at developing new drugs; in 2018 another six or so failed to meet the mark. Some drugs are discontinued their trails. The latest exciting news is medication that will radically delay or maybe even stop the development of the condition. Needless to say, this would change the future of every affected person and their families.

How to Strive in the Shadow of Alzheimer's is a new book by Jamie Tyrone, a woman with a super-rare genetic predisposition for Alzheimer's that affects only 2% of the population. Marwan Sabbagh, director of Cleveland Clinic's Lou Ruvo Center for Brain Health, details Jamie's remarkable journey from misdiagnosis to diagnosis, from despair to determination, as she joined forces with Sabbagh to fight for her brain health. From her story come surefire ways that you can protect your brain so that you may never develop dementia, delay its onset, or slow its progress.

Alzheimer's Disease includes high blood pressure, diabetes, high (LDL) cholesterol, and vascular disease. Optimizing health conditions has a downstream benefit of reducing risk for developing Alzheimer's Disease:

They are . . . women with type 2 Diabetes. The risk is even higher if they have genetic predisposition (ApoE4). Obesity, that causes visceral fat around the belly and triggers a 72% increase in dementia risk. Smoke, which develops AD eight years earlier than nonsmokers.[343]

You can avoid all the above by: 1) adopting a healthy diet, such as blends of the Mediterranean and DASH diets, rich in B complex, fruits, and vegetables high vitamin C, and unsaturated fat and spices; 2) getting regular physical exercise a minimum of 30 minutes daily, at least five days a week, plus resistance exercises; 3) tamping down your stress (highly inflammatory) with daily moving and mindful meditations, and participating in religious activities, and 4) involving yourself in volunteer activities, putting others' needs ahead of your own.

To find quality physical and emotional support, check out the Alzheimer's Association (alz.org), or the National Institute on Aging (nia.nih.gov). Appendix E has a list of other resources.

15

Helping Caregivers and Families Cope with Their Responsibilities

> All caregivers need hope . . . hope perhaps from an informed theological perspective that provides a sense of purpose in the face of the injury, hope perhaps from the therapist that sees return of function not just adaptation as a feasible treatment goal, or perhaps hope in the form of someone willing to simply listen, to get into the deep water with us; these are examples of the real "cup of cold water" needed that bond us to professionals of all disciplines.[344]

According to the AARP, more than five million older persons in U.S. require some types of assisted living to keep them to be independent. Contrary to popular opinion, most American families do not abandon family members with disabilities, diseases, and conditions to paid professionals and paraprofessionals. Instead, the families play the central role in extending health care service. Most caregivers either come from elderly spouses and/or adult children. Older adult caregivers, often with their own physical ailments or disability, frequently experience greater emotional and physical stress because of the heavy responsibilities they must shoulder. For caregivers of person who have dementia or

Alzheimer's disease, the burden of care is even greater. From early to later stages, the demand for care of the demented person is enormous.

Particularly in the latter stage, the demented person requires 24-hour supervision, causing caregivers sleep deprivation at night and fatigue throughout the day. Thus, caregivers easily become socially isolated and do not have time to nurture relationships with others. Due to all the problems and tasks they are required to perform 24/7 to care for the demented person, with some degree of guilt many end up placing their loved one in nursing homes as the final resort to keep them in sane.[345] It is not all surprising that depression, anxiety, trouble sleeping, marital conflict, alcohol use, and medical illness are all higher among caregivers.[346]

Holly Gershbein and Lauren Austin, authors of the book, *Love, Loss and Dementia*, want caregivers to know that others understand what they are going through, especially those caring for loved one with dementia. They are not alone, they are not losing their minds, and they will survive. Yes, there will be times of stress, feelings of isolation, loneliness, continual guilt, helplessness, and mental and emotional exhaustion. This journey is not easy, but it is a labor of love. When caregivers say goodbye to their loved one with dementia, they will grieve but will heal. This is the message that the authors want to convey. "Unless one has been there, caring for a loved one with this disease, it is hard to understand all that caregivers go through, and the mental and physical exhaustion can take a toll on a family," Gershbein said.[347]

When Gershbein was going through this with her mother, she not only kept a journal, but she also read everything she could find about the disease. When she did not find anything to help her, to help her understand what she was going through, she and Lauren wrote a book to help others going through it. There is a host of information on Alzheimer and dementia on the National Institute of Aging's website, www.nia.nih. gov. Also see the author explaining what Alzheimer's disease is and the distinction between natural aging and Alzheimer in detail. Alzheimer is not a part of aging.

As stated, there is no cure for Alzheimer's disease. Some sources, however, claim that products such as coconut oil or dietary supplements such as Protandim can cure or delay it, but there is no scientific evidence to support these claims. There are several drugs approved by USFDA to treat the symptoms of the disease. Certain medications and other approaches can help control behavioral symptoms. Currently, there is no definitive evidence about what can prevent the disease or age-related cognitive decline. What we know is that a healthy life style—one that includes a healthy diet, physical activity, appropriate weight control, and no smoking can lower the risk of certain chronic diseases and boost overall health and wellbeing. The best chance anyone has is to maintain a healthy lifestyle to delay, slow down, or even prevent the disease, as well as social and religious activity and intellectual stimulation for those at risk for Alzheimer's.

"My mother needed round-the-clock care and financially we could not handle the expenses. So we placed my mother in a nursing home where she would have the care she needed," Gershbein said. People say her book validates what they are going through, and find the comfort in knowing someone understands and has already walked this difficult path. "My mother has been gone for four years, and we decided to write this book to help others that are on this journey. We want caregivers to know they are not alone, and others have and will walk in their shoes," Gershbein said. Looking back, she sees there are so many things they should have done differently, the first of which is to be good to yourself and take care of yourself.

Caregiver Stress

Many caregivers for those with Alzheimer's and other dementias experience significant stress, which can put their own health at risk. To assess a caregiver's stress level and get resources to help, Alzheimer's Association has provided, *Caregiver Stress Check* at alz.org/care, or follow the tips below:

1. Contact your local Alzheimer's Association chapter to learn about resources available in your community.

2. Further your knowledge about Alzheimer's disease and caregiving techniques by attending workshops or by going to alz.org/care.
3. Get help from family, friends, and community resources.
4. Accept changes as they occur.
5. Be realistic about what you can manage.
6. Keep current with doctor appointments.
7. Take care of yourself by watching your diet, exercising, and getting plenty of rest.
8. Make legal and financial plans.
9. Give yourself credit for what you has accomplished. Don't feel guilty if you lose patience or can't do everything on your own.

Besides the above, there are many things pastoral caregivers can do to help to relieve the burden of those who must care for chronically ill or demented family members. These include providing:

1. *Respite from caregiving responsibilities.* Church members and pastors may take turns spending times with the patient, thus allowing caregivers some time for themselves. Larger churches may sponsor an adult day care that provides structural activities for demented persons. Some privately-run day care programs may exist in the community. The church and congregation can provide financial help to offset the care expenses. In-home patient sitting is another option.
2. *Companionship and social outlets.* Simply being a friend and companion to the caregiver can relieve the stress of caregiving and help combat the isolation. Chat on the phone, visit the caregiver's home, take them to movie or dinner, or arrange for the caregiver to participate in social activities, either in the church or community. Be friends with them, a role that members of a church congregation can often fulfill. Most importantly, they must be motivated, know of the need, and realize how important it is to provide such companionship.
3. *Practical help.* Do whatever you can to help to relieve some of the caregiver's responsibilities—provide transportation for doctor's

appointments, cook meals for them often, do yard work, clean the house for them, do repair work, and so on.

4. *Counseling and spiritual support.* Simply talking about their stress to a concerned pastor and train counselor can help caregivers feel less isolated and alone when depression and anxiety impairs their functioning. Of primary importance is encouraging spiritually and showing caregivers how to rely on their religious faith and relationship with God to cope with the situation.[348]

5. *Information and Education.* Pastoral counselors can help caregivers find the necessary resources and information that can help them achieve some control over their situation. Pastoral counselors need to be sensitive to how much information the caregiver wants and needs at any point in the patient's illness. Caregiver support groups exist in most communities, the participation in which helps the caregiver to counteract social isolation and provide a forum for sharing experiences. If qualified, pastoral counselors can help with legal matters (or facilitate with someone knowledgeable)—will, living will, power of attorney, and so on.

6. *Permission for replacement.* Clergy and physicians are in an ideal position to "give permission" to relieve caregiver's guilt feeling and ease them to continue to minister to and spend time with a relative once the person is placed into the nursing home.

7. *Small Group Ministry.* Pastor and pastoral staff such as counselors cannot do all the ministry, counseling, emotional support, and fulfillment of other needs that older or chronically ill persons have. Small groups, however, each consisting of about ten older and younger persons, can be created within the church.[349] As approved by the pastor, volunteer group leaders and their home or other groups could meet once a week and offer several functions—Bible study, prayer, fellowship, and meals. These small groups serve two functions: First, use of their talents and gifts to serve the needs of others in their home group. Second, serve in reducing the isolation and loneliness of their members. In this way, ministry to older adults is spread throughout the church body.

Four-Step Plan to Help Prepare for When
Your Loved One Needs a Caregiver

There comes a time when we realize no matter how independent our loved one is, they are going to need help as they get older. Around 20 million or more Americans currently are providing care for aging parents or elder relatives, according to AARP and the National Alliance for Caregiving's statistics. How do you plan ahead for such a big unknown? Los Angeles-based geriatric care consultant, Jennifer Voorles, says, "So many families avoid talking about this until something happens, but it's much more difficult to make decisions in a crisis." The following four steps—where, who, how, and what—will help guide you to the right path.

1. Consider **Where** (living options). Senior living today has come a long way from the nursing homes of old—ranging from retirement enclaves to tiered continuing care retirement communities offering a variety of levels of assistances. Yet "aging in place" is by far the most popular option. A full 95% of Americans age 65 and older say they want and wish to remain in their home. Loved ones should consider how mobility issues or chronic conditions—both of which are likely to get more serious with time—might affect what kind of care they may need. Therefore, it is never too early to consult with a geriatric professionals who can help to assess the senior's needs, weigh options, and find resources. Check with employment assistance programs such as elder care, offering various location services, access to legal advice, and other assistance. Use the Aging Life Care Association's search referral to find a qualified local expert.

2. Consider **Who** (assess caregiving availability). Approximate 89% of all long-term care in the U.S. is provided free by family members. It may be too early for you and your family members (siblings) to decide who will be doing what, but you can discuss how everyone's location, job, and family obligations will factor in, says Gail Gibson Hunt, founder of the *National Alliance for Caregiving*. Do this via family meeting or conference calls, and

ask everyone to be as honest as possible about their capabilities. In many cases, siblings come up with creative ways to balance responsibilities, assigning more of the financial burden to siblings who live at a distance or have more demanding careers, and more of the hands-on help to those who live closer or have more flexible work situations. Remember that the amount of help needed likely will increase, says Voorlas. "This situation could go on for many years, and ones often don't know if it's going to be a temporary crisis or if it's just beginning of a step-down decline."[350] Plan to revisit the sharing of responsibilities regularly so that no one sibling ends up stressed and overwhelmed.

3. Consider **How** (handling finances). Just 7.2 million Americans have long-term care policies, according to AARP survey data. On average, caregivers spend $7,000 a year out of pocket caring for a loved one. The good news is that there are many sources of financial help. If either of the seniors are pension-eligible veterans, for example, VA programs, under certain circumstances, will pay for residential and in-home care. Life insurance policies can be accelerated to pay living benefits, or cashed out. On the state and local level, subsidized transportation, meal and day-care activity programs can be a lifeline for family caregivers stretched to the max. While money and end-of-life care are not exactly fun dinner-table topics, caregiving will be much less stressful with at least some of these decisions already in place. Seniors need time to get used to the idea, but making sure their wishes are heard will help ease the way.[351]

4. Consider **What** (protecting financial future). Alzheimer's strips individuals of their cognitive and physical abilities, leaving caregivers to make decisions on finances, healthcare, and other important matters. While the numbers are daunting, taking the four steps below now can help protect your own and your loved one's financial future.

1) *Prepare for health costs.* Most people are not prepared to pay for the large financial burden of dementia related illnesses.

However, it is one can do before a diagnosis is given. Between 2000-2050, the out of pocket costs for caring a demented person and his family is projected to grow by 400 %. Reviewing now for all possible financial sources (insurance plan, and adjusting based on how one feel would best suite one's needs.

2) *Formalize advanced directives.* There are two advanced directives: 1) Living will—affirms a person's choices for future medical care decisions and wishes by allowing them to state their wishes regarding their health care and end-of-life decisions while they are still thinking clearly. Caretakers can be confident that their loved one is continuing to live as they planned. 2) Durable power of attorney—allows a caretaker to make financial, medical, and other decisions, consistent with the person's wishes, on behalf of the individual. You should always consult with your legal advisor or attorney to discuss the need for and details of wills and power of attorney.

3) *Discuss finances.* Loved ones should discuss finances and bank accounts while the individual's cognitive abilities are least impaired. These critical discussions help loved ones ensure that finances are preserved for continued care and are not subject to unscrupulous swindles.

4) *Financial independence.* Since the disease has robbed individuals of their freedom, if still appropriate, allow them to continue to pay bills and have their own spending money to create a sense of self-sufficiency. Give them a sense of autonomy by setting up auto-pay for many bills.

Nearly half of American over the age of 85 have Alzheimer's today, which makes it critical for us to be aware of the symptoms and what to do in the wake of diagnosis to help minimize the emotional impact of diagnosis, and to reach out to legal and financial advisors to help ensure personal affairs are in order.[352]

The Character of the Caregiver

The great and complex challenges of the onset of dementia become a day of reckoning within a family and for all concerned. The character of the caregiver plays a vital role in dementia. As the author of *The Alzheimer's Sourcebook for Caregivers* has observed, "If we do not deal with our own issue of love and grief around the failures of love, we cannot live with Alzheimer's disease."[353] It is as if we need all of our own life, in all maturation and fruition, to stand up to the final test of our own personal resources and meet the challenges we will face with the dementia of our loved one. How do we love the "no goes" (undisciplined or unchurched people) in our congregation and families?

Thus the onset of dementia may also induce a bio-psycho-social spiritual crisis within the inner lives of family members who now are faced with unprecedented emotional challenges. The emotional life of the demented is heightened with uninhibited bouts of frustration, anger, fear, and loss of significance and identity. The natural response of caregivers often will be negative instead of positive. Coming to terms with the illness may be a long, slow process requiring growing understanding and patience. This is the time when the church could lead the way in helping its members lovingly prepare for the care of aging parents, rather than simply reacting to the crisis.[354] Such preparation might shore-up scriptural admonitions to honor fathers and mothers. "No goes" provide the family and the church with an opportunity to learn how to love in ways that are able to meet the most difficult of tests. This also helps caregivers to learn to depend upon the Holy Spirit for the capacity to love in a Christian manner. All positive responses are summed-up in one concluding need—*love*—which is unpacked in the following five basic needs of human personhood:

Comfort. Our first instinct is to whisper comfort to the loved one who is beginning to lose coping abilities. Comfort provides inner strength when their world is falling apart. The emotional life becomes raw and the oscillations of anger and distrust create swinging moods of strong dialectics. This can change like a storm on a placid lake suddenly and unexpectedly. The person is struggling to remain a person despite their disability. The sense of loss requires empathy and immediate response of support in sudden moments of personal loss.

Attachment. The medical pronouncement, "The patient has Alzheimer's" is like the pronouncement of, "They have leprosy." There is the immediate feeling of separation, of distancing your own cognitive skills from the one now going "crazy," and you become sensitive to the slightest sense of being now somewhat separate. Thus, there is a deepening sense of being cut-off from your loved one, and of new threats of loneliness, which underscores the importance of attachment as a vital gift of the caregiver. Attachment implies the vital need of bonding, as is most often discussed with respect to childhood. "A need of a child to be bonded can be extended to explain the ongoing importance of baby-boomers throughout life."[355] People with dementia are continually finding themselves in situations they experience as strange. Providing a familiar and consistent environment that includes the underlying loyalty of the caregiver allows the senior to remain stronger in spirit.

Inclusion. This involves our intrinsic need of belonging, of not being exiled and alone.

We are created to be social beings, "made in the image and likeness of God." Having close family ties and living in community should be norms of personhood. Individualism itself is a cultural deficiency, not a human benefit. Those with dementia feel the threat of being cut-off as sensitively as those who are deaf or blind. Thus, the more deterioration that sets in, the more they seek attention. In the past, this need was not met, and seniors often were left terribly alone. This is the "bubble of isolation" in which seniors with advanced dementia can dwell.[356] When such needs for inclusion are not met, the downwards spiral may quickly end in death. But in reverse, when treated as a person, the senior may once more have hope and be given space and dignity.

Occupation. As in the novel, *Still Alice*, as soon as she was diagnosed with Alzheimer's disease, she has to quit her prestigious professorship. It is all over? she wonders. In actuality, occupation is more than ones job. It reflects upon our significance in many different ways. Gradual relinquishment is kinder, more affirming, and therapeutic. When we are deprived suddenly of our accustomed occupations, we atrophy in our giftedness. Caregivers must know seniors well enough to know what gives the deepest satisfaction and sense of significance.

Identity. We all have a name that distinguishes us from others. This mirror our need to have a unique identity, which is also our narrative, our story, which make us unique, giving unity and meaning to our continued existence. This link, between past and future, gives, courage to face the unknown future even in the presence of death. Our birthday and family lore have placed us within a specific set of relationships. It becomes crucial with dementia to know that even when we may forget our own identity, with memories fading away about many things, we are not forgotten, for others now hold our memory instead as loving recorders of our past. Caregivers who take the time to learn about the personal history of dementia sufferers, or friends and family members who can play a part in recalling the life stories of those to whom they provide companionship and care, offer a great care gift to those whose self-identity is in peril.

If caregivers are able to imagine themselves to be the sufferers, they could express more empathy to respond more easily to meeting the needs of the sufferers. Yet the natural reactions of caregivers commonly contribute the opposite toward these primary needs. The wounds of the demented wound them as well, as if the caregiver needed the most comfort. The human response is to feel more repulsed when kind intentions are misunderstood, and then anger alienates caregivers and the demented further. Caregivers often interpret their roles as requiring them to take charge and "do the job properly," which only generates more helplessness for the sufferer of dementia. This results in a further sense of worthlessness and a further loss of personal identity for the victim of dementia, which further spirals downward into depression and even deeper alienation.

16

Current Developments in
Treating Alzheimer's Disease

For years, doctors believed that growing new brain cells was impossible, and we would always be defenseless against these horrible diseases. *As it turns out, they were wrong.*

No matter how old we are, we CAN regenerate neurons. This is because of a special compound known as *nerve growth factor—NGF* for short. We can think of it as the energy source our brain needs to grow and replenish itself. When we are young, our levels of NGF are high. So our brains are constantly forming plump new neurons, bursting at the seams with neurotransmitters. At the same time, NGF is helping our neurons create dense networks of communication lines, called axons, that help them transmit messages between each other.

In a healthy brain, there are more than 100 trillion of these connections, sending lifesaving signals back and forth every single day. To put that in perspective, an Olympic-sized swimming pool can hold roughly 200 billion grains of sand. If you were to take that swimming pool and multiply it by 500 . . . that is how many connections there are in your brain.

As well, it takes a lot of NGF to maintain that operation. But unfortunately, like the gas tank in your car, your NGF eventually runs out. When that happens your brains loses the ability to make new neural cells.

But good news—a mysterious food from the mountainous Nara Prefecture of Japan can "refill the tank" of your brain's NGF.

Yamabushitake Regeneration

The isolated monks who wander the mountain forests here call this mysterious brain tonic "Yamabushitake," which they have used for thousands of years to increase their mental clarity, focus, and as a meditation aid. Now, trial after trial is showing that this ancient wisdom has the potential to stop and even reverse neurodegenerative disease.

Two incredible compounds within the Yamabushitake actually replenish our body's natural NGF tank, so that all of a sudden, our brain is flooded with waves of replenishing nerve growth factor that immediately rebuilds our neurons. This lays new connections between our brain cells, and supports the production of memory-boosting neurotransmitters. In a sense, it is like our brains are aging in reverse.

Already, more than a dozen clinical trials have shown the "Yamabushitake" to be near miraculous in its ability to regrow brain cells. Clinical trials done at the Institute of Biological Sciences demonstrated that Yamabushitake could regenerate neurons by as much as 60%, with as much as 22% of that regeneration seen in just 48 hours.[357]

When Japanese researchers tested these effects on a large group of 50- to 80-year-old patients, all of them were cognitively impaired, they found that the Yamabushitake erased years of mental decline. It was an incredible result, but the powers of Yamabushitake do not stop there. In patients with Alzheimer's, sticky molecules known as beta-amyloids form together in clumps and attach themselves to neurons. They cut off the blood supply to whichever brain cell to which they are connected, effectively suffocating it until it withers and dies. Needless to say, we want to stay as far away from these nasty compounds as possible, which is why the Yamabushitake is so amazing. It forms a protective force field around your neurons that lets nourishing nutrients in, but keeps the brain-killing beta-amyloids from touching your brain cells.

In this way, your neurons, and the connections between them, stay pristine. Now, patients can use the Yamabushitake from the comfort of their own home to help their brain regrow and regenerate itself. They do not have to go to a doctor's office or deal with an insurance company. Of course, individual results vary, but it has been shown to dramatically improve brain health in just two days. Anything that promising surely deserves a shot, but it comes with a warning: You have to get the right form of Yamabushitake for it to work. The compounds inside it first have to be extracted and then activated through a two-step process.

Unfortunately, most of the Yamabushitake on the market is only extracted but not activated, so your body cannot use it. You might as well be throwing your money in the trash can. In fact, eBay is the only one place known of where you can get Yamabushitake that has been properly extracted and activated so it preserves all of the beneficial, brain-revitalizing compounds for maximum NGF production.

Will There Soon Be a Cure for Alzheimer's?

Impressive new research led by scientists from UT Southwestern discovered the earliest point in the neurodegenerative process that is thought to lead to dementia. The researchers described their discovery like finding the "Big Bang" of Alzheimer's disease, and they hope that their work leads to new treatments and ways to detect the disease before major symptoms occur. Marc Diamond, a primary collaborator on this new study, says that "this is perhaps the biggest finding we have made to date, though it will likely be some time before any benefits materialize in the clinic. This changes much of how we think about the problem."[358]

Modern Alzheimer's research usually concentrates on a specific protein called Amyloid Beta, mentioned above, and the clumping of that protein is suspected to be the primary pathological cause of the disease's symptoms. After a long series of clinical trial failures in drugs designed to attack these amyloid beta plaques, however, some scientists are turning their attention elsewhere. New research focuses on a different protein that is called "tau." These tau proteins have been found to form abnormal clumps in the brain, called "neurofibrillary tangles," which accumulate and kill neurons. Some researchers have hypothesized that this is the primary cause of Alzheimer's.

Until now, it was not known how or when these tau proteins began to accumulate into tangles in the brain. It was previously believed that isolated tau proteins did not have a distinctly harmful shape until they began to aggregate with other tau proteins, but this new research has shown that a toxic tau protein actually presents itself as misfolded, exposing parts that are usually folded inside, before it begins to aggregate. It is these exposed parts of the protein that enable aggregation, forming the larger toxic tangles.

Diamond says that "we think of this as the 'Big Bang' of tau pathology. This is a way of peering to the very beginning of the disease process. It moves us back to a very discreet point where we see the appearance of the first molecular change that leads to neurodegeneration in Alzheimer's."[359]

From here, the research is due to take two separate prospective pathways. First, researchers will look at developing a simple diagnostic test to detect signs of this abnormal tau protein, either by taking a blood sample or a spinal fluid test. If these toxic tau proteins can be easily detected, then doctors might be able to diagnose Alzheimer's before the major degenerative symptoms have taken hold. Second, research involves investigating prospective drug treatments that could interrupt the tau aggregation process. The researchers point to a new drug called "Tafamidis" as an example of a medicine that was designed to stabilize a protein that can clump and cause adverse symptoms.

Tafamidis was created to delay impairment to nerve function caused by the toxic accumulation of a normally harmless protein called transthyretin, which currently is approved for use in Europe and Japan. The FDA, however, has called for further clinical proof before this drug is available for use in the U.S. Now that this early alteration in the shape of tau molecules has been identified, researchers can focus on potential drug targets to inhibit the toxic accumulation at this stage. "The hunt is on to build on this finding and make a treatment that blocks the neurodegeneration process where it begins. If it works, the incidence of Alzheimer's disease could be substantially reduced," says Diamond.[360]

As shown, there are several new research and development efforts currently being conducted all around the world, some of which have good results and others not so much, but there is a realistic hope that one day the treatment of and possible cure will be realized—through God's intervention—sooner rather than later.

Note: So many more new researches to find treatment and cure of this disease have been conducted in all around the world in recent years, author are unable to enlist all of them. Readers are argued readers — for their own benefits do their own research to know more about this disease.

17

Conclusion

It is undeniable that dementia, the Alzheimer's disease in particular, is a terrible disease. This cruel disease not only steals one's memories and independence, but it finally steals one's dignity by eroding the ability to manage the basic tasks of daily life. In short, it steals one's personhood. This disease progresses slowly and often cannot be diagnosed early, but the most tragic reality is it has no cure for now.

How can this disease of Alzheimer's, a dementia, be developed to have a theological perspective in the core of Christian praxis? Such a perspective takes a serious established knowledge, and seeks to enable the discovery of options, possibilities, and perspectives that are not available from other sources of knowledge, but which are crucial for a truly Christian understanding of dementia and the development of authentically Christian modes of dementia care. Medicine may not use theology to bring cure of a person with dementia, *but it may help people to cope better with suffering.* What is rarely considered is the fact that the goal of medicine and theology and their respective definitions of health and wellbeing may be significantly different. Grafting theology into the goal of medicine on the grounds of its potential therapeutic benefit could lead to confusion, dissonance, distortion, and contradiction. Wellbeing within Christianity is not gauged by the presence or absence of illness or distress. Religious beliefs and practices may well have therapeutic benefit but that is not their primary function or intention.

Theologically speaking, wellbeing has nothing to do with the absence or reduction of anything. It has to do with the presence of something: the presence of God-in-relationship. Wellbeing, peace, health—what Scripture describes as *shalom* (a more complex word than peace)—has to do with the presence of a specific God who engages in personal relationships with unique individuals for formative purposes understood in redemptive and relational terms. This is not to suggest that there cannot and should not be a creative and healing conversation between medicine and theology. Rather, theology provides an understanding of the basic context into which medical sciences speak, especially given the understanding that medicine is practiced within the context of creation and under the providential sovereignty of God. In a real sense, "neurology is theology"; thus, the dementia is a thoroughly theological condition. Many verses in the Bible offer comfort and peace to sufferers of the disease and to those who are caregivers or providers, under any circumstances at any time.

The author has tried his best to present an overall positive, fair, honest, hopeful, and challenging perspective on Alzheimer's in different lights, and to describe it in a fresh way from a theological perspective. Dementia may be a tragic affliction, but there is much to be hoped for as long as we can establish the types of relationship and communities that will allow us to perceive the disease properly and realistically. As we remember our loved ones with dementia as God does, may it drive our presence into their presence. No matter how much a person might try to redescribe dementia, the elements of pain, tragedy, and affliction cannot be avoided or written out of the story. Healing begins with an honest acknowledgement of the truth. Only when we recognize the pain of dementia can the things that the author has offered begin to make sense and initiate change. The sadness of dementia need not, and indeed must not, be allowed to have the final word. Even in the midst of pain and affliction that can accompany dementia, there are hidden possibilities if we trust God and allow the challenge of our sadness to stimulate new ways of thinking and being with one another.

A number of important practices highlighted here have potential to bring us out of the brokenness of dementia:

- Critical thinking and re-description
- Care and reflection of godly action
- Recognition of holiness in the other
- Presence and being with the other
- Remembering well
- Lament
- Hospitality among strangers
- Visitation

At the heart of these practices is "visitation." If we do not take time to visit one another, do not take time to be present for one another, we will never see Alzheimer's for what it really is. Therefore, we must visit one another—spend time together and offer friendship, respite, relief, listening, and loving presence to both sufferers and caregivers. We must give people with dementia the benefit of the doubt, and not allow the stories that we assume to be so convincing to prevent us from seeing the face of Jesus in these struggling ones. As we practice these things in these ways, God is worshipped and attended to. In the end, a little piece of heaven is revealed on earth.

Many think Matthew 6:10 is a prayer for the future; it is not. We can experience something of heaven here on earth. When God's will is done, then heaven is revealed. When we care for others and act in accordance with our renewed vision, we come to see God more clearly and act more faithfully. Heaven is truly in our hearts, even when on our hearts are afflicted and broken. We are remembered and lifted up by the words in the book of Deuteronomy, "Be strong and courageous! Do not be afraid and do not panic before them. For the Lord your God will personally go ahead of you. He will neither fail you nor forsake you" (Deut. 31:6). When we encounter dementia in others or ourselves, we can find solace and hope in Jesus and in his words: "Be sure of this: *I am with you always, even to the end of the earth.*" In any circumstance, these promises are felt, touched, and lived into truth. May Thy will be Done on Earth as It is in Heaven.

APPENDIX A

Types of Dementia

From the core definition, dementia is a brain disease, the product of brain damage brought on by a variety of difference causes. A series of subcategories of dementia are worked out based on various causal factors.

Alzheimer's Disease. During the cause of the disease, the chemistry and structure of the brain changes, leading to the death of brain cells.

Vascular Dementia. The oxygen supply to the brain falls and brain cells may die. The symptoms can occur either suddenly, following a stroke, or over time, through a series of small strokes.

Dementia with Lewy Bodies. Gets its name from tiny spherical structures that develop inside nerve cells. Their presence in the brain leads to the degeneration of brain tissue.

Fronto-Temporal Dementia. Damage is usually focused in the front part of the brain. Personality and behavior are initially more affected than memory.

Korsakoff's Syndrome. A brain disorder that is usually associated with heavy drinking over a long period. Although it is not, strictly speaking, a dementia, people with the condition experience loss of short-term memory.

Creuzfeldt-Jokob Disease. Prions are infectious agents that attack the central nervous system and then invade the brain, causing dementia. The best example of prion disease is Creuzfeldt-Jokob Disease, or CJD.

HIV-related Cognitive Impairment. People with AIDs and HIV sometimes develop cognitive impairment, particularly in the later stages of their illness.

Mild Cognitive Impairment. MCI is a relatively recent term used to describe people who have some problems with their memory but do not actually have dementia.

Rare Causes of Dementia.[361] This includes progressive supranuclear palsy and Binswanger's disease. People with multiple sclerosis, motor neuron disease, Parkinson's disease, or Huntington's disease are at increased risk of developing dementia.

There is strong evidence yet that the herpes virus is a cause of Alzheimer's, suggesting that effective and safe antiviral drugs might be able to treat the disease. The virus implicated in Alzheimer's disease, herpes simplex virus type 1 (HSV1), is better known for causing cold sores in many elderly people. HSV1 is also present in the brain of those who have a specific gene known as APOE4. Currently, several medicines are in the developmental stage.

APPENDIX B

Choosing a Nursing Home

"Choose my instruction instead of silver, knowledge rather than choice gold." (Proverbs 8:10)

I have visited several nursing facilities in Houston City area. I also spent more than two years as a volunteer at assisted living facilities in the city. Following is my observation: Nearly 45% of all people reaching the age 65 will enter a nursing home at some time in their lives (Kemper and Murtaugh 1991); however, only about 5% of old persons are actually living in these setting at any one time. It is an extremely stressful and painful experience, both for the older adults and family caregivers to place a loved one in a nursing home. To make this transition as easy as possible, pastor or counselors can provide information about when nursing home placement has become necessary, availability of other types of living arrangements, and how to choose a nursing home. As well, they can help inform regarding responsibilities family members will have soon after the placement has taken place:

1. *When placement become necessary.* Generally, it is better for older persons to be cared for in their own homes because nursing houses often are short-staffed and underpaid. Therefore, nursing homes provide care that is less than optimal. Nevertheless, there are still a few good homes that provide adequate care. It becomes an excellent solution, especially if family members are able to involve themselves in the patient's care in the nursing home. To

care for patients in their own home, supervision and safety are of prime importance as well as available time that caregivers can devote to caring for the patient. Some patients may require 24/7 care, which also needs to be considered by caregivers. One more reason to decide on a nursing home is if the care demands of the patient are too complex or too great to be met by the caregivers (professional or family members) in the home setting, or the cost of home care becomes too great to be met.

2. *Alternative living arrangements.* Depending on the level of care the patient requires, there may be other options, including the following:

   a. Condominiums
   b. Shared housing
   c. Home sharing
   d. Rental apartments
   e. Subsidized
   f. Continuing Care Communities (Life Care Communities)
   g. Independent and assisted-living retirement communities

The following are types of 24/7 care. They are institutional settings that vary depending on the amount of nursing care required by the elder:

   h. Adult foster care homes
   i. Rest homes (domiciliary care)
   j. Family care home
   k. Home for the aged
   l. Nursing homes (intermediate care, ICF)
   m. Nursing homes (skilled care, SNF)
   n. Special care units

Five basic criteria need to be considered in choosing a nursing home:

1. The cost
2. Reputation in the community

3. Location
4. Staffing

Also helpful is the publication, "Guide to Choosing a Nursing Home," by the U.S. Department of Health and Human Services publication #HCFA-02174 (1993).

Family responsibilities after placement include managing beside resentment from the elder, assisting in their adjustment of the new living arrangement, and addressing the guilty feelings of the family members who place the elder in the nursing home. Both patient and family sides of the situation require intervention. Clergy and pastoral counselors are in ideal positions to help. Visitation and counseling to both elderly and family members often are inevitable to resolve the different feelings from both elderly and family members. When it becomes necessary, some type of guidance should be sought.

A major reason for facilitating reconciliation is to clear the air so that family members will visit and spend time with the elder in the nursing home. Besides assuring that adequate care is received, their visits will help relieve the loneliness and isolation that the elder may experience in this setting. Since between 50% to 75% of nursing residents have dementia, mentally alert elders suffer the most in these settings because they have relatively few persons with whom they can relate. Instead, they end up depending heavily on family members to provide them with social interaction and support. Pastoral counselors and church members can play a major role as surrogate family for these persons by providing monthly visits for counseling, prayer, or receiving Communion. Weekly visits by clergy, members of the congregation, or children can do wonders to reduce the elders' isolation and give them a sense of being care for. At the same time, such activities help the elder find purpose and meaning in their new life by contributing to the lives of others at the nursing home.[362]

Even elders with severe memory impairment and advanced Alzheimer's disease retain the capacity to experience emotion. They sense the caring and kindness, or the lack of it, of those around them. Anyone can minister to severely demented elders by showing concern and care, praying for them, laying hands on them while praying, reading the Bible to them, or singing old hymns to and with them. These are the sick person that Jesus calls us to visit and care for, and when we do so, we minister to Christ himself (Matthew 25:39–40).

APPENDIX C

Community Resources for Older Persons

"Love your neighbor as yourself." (Leviticus 19:18)

There are many community resources that may help older persons remain living independently in their homes or make the burden of caregiving in the home easier. The list of types of community resources available—from the NC Division of Aging, 1995—can be uploaded from https://www.nsdhhs.gov.divisions/daas. Also available is a "North Carolina Caregiver's Handbook," by the NC Department of Human Resources, Division of Aging, 1995.

Pastoral counselors also can call the local area agency on aging. The following government-sponsored programs are devoted to providing for the needs of the elderly in particular regions:

• Alliance for Mentally Ill	800-451-9682
• National Hospice Organization	800-658-8898
• Senior Health Insurance Information	800-443-9354
• Social Security Administration	800-7721213
• Social Security/SSI Disability Hot Line	800-638-6310

Furthermore, there are resources available for Alzheimer's Disease is diagnosed as follows:

- Alzheimer's Disease and related Dementia and related Dementia Education and Referral Center (ADEAR) — 800-438-4380
- Alzheimer's Disease Research (ADR) — 855-345-6237
- ARCH National Respite Network — 703-256-2084
- Care Pathways — 877-521-9987
- Caregiver Resource Center — 203-861-9833
- Family Caregiver Alliance — 800-445-8106
- Home Instead Senior Care — 888-330-8210
- Leading Age — 202-783-2242
- Medicare — 800-633-4227
- National Adult Day Services association — 877-745-1440
- National Caregivers Library — 804-327-1111
- National Center for Assisted Living — 202-842-4444
- National Hospice and Palliative Care Organization — 703-837-1500
- National Long Term Care Ombudsman Resource Center — 202-332-2275
- Social Security Administration — 800-772-1213

APPENDIX D

Expanded Views on Dementia
by Kitwood and Sabat

Both Kitwood and Sabat want to expand the definition of what dementia is to include the significance of such things as love, relationships, and care. This, I have argued, is a much stronger and more appropriate place for theology and pastoral care to begin the journey into dementia. We begin by thinking through the implications of Kitwood's suggestion that dementia has to do with relational disorders and his attempts to develop what he describes as a "neurology of personhood,"[363] that is, a model of what he describes as a personhood that recognizes and seeks to bring to the fore the intimate connection between neurology and social experience.

Challenging the Standard Paradigm

The heart of Kitwood's project is his desire to persuade health and social care services to recognize the personhood of people with dementia and to provide a firm practical and theoretical foundation that will open up the possibility of caregivers engaging in forms of personal relationships that are not unnecessarily influenced by the tendency toward Imperfectionism. He describes the established medical approach to dementia as "the standard paradigm."[364] The approach has emerged from classical science, which says that there is a straightforward, linear connection between brain pathology and the behaviors and experiences that someone chooses to name as dementia. The pattern moves from causal phenomena to neuropathic change to dementia.[365] The progression is linear, moving from brain pathology (neurological damage, malfunction, or deficit, disease, genetics, and so forth) directly to the manifestations of the symptom of dementia. All of this remains internal to the individual's brain. Dementia thus is located firmly within individual selves. Standard procedures designed to describe, identify, and treat the condition of dementia are then applied based on the understand that they are dealing with specifically neurological conditions that have some forms of identifiable biological basis and which, in principle, are open up neurological, pharmacological, or genetic intervention. Kitwood notes,

> There are many allowable variants in the paradigm and controversies among investigators about the details of the process they postulate. The aim is to identify the X (causal factors) as a set of necessary conditions, together with the precise causal mechanism . . . in genetic research, the ultimate aim is to remove X altogether. In all of this the basic linear sequence remain largely unchallenged.[366]

Within the paradigm, human beings with dementia live in a social context rather than as isolated monads that are presumed to be unimportant for understanding the key elements of what dementia is and how it should be responded to. Kitwood notices that the standard paradigm has significant flaws despite how influential it has been. Three problematic areas in particular have been identified:

1. *The lack of continuity between the level of neurological damage and manifestation of dementia.* In some cases, people have gone through the manifestations of dementia only to have it discovered that they do not have more neurological damage than a person of similar age without the manifestations of dementia.[367] This to suggest that the initial diagnosis was flawed. In other words, those who adhere strictly to the standard paradigm when faced

with challenges are not to question the paradigm but to assume the phenomenon was mistakenly included and needs to be placed in a different category. Kitwood argues that there may be a different and more radical explanation.

2. *The issue of rapid decline.* A well-documented observation is that "some people with dementia, under certain conditions, deteriorate in their functioning very much faster than can be attributed to the consequence of progressive degeneration of nerve tissue."[368] For instance, when a person with dementia loses a loved one or is taken out of their familiar environment such as home and placed in a care facility, it is common that they move quickly into a more advanced stage of dementia. If dementia has a natural history that is bound by a flexible theory of inevitable neurological decline that progresses through recognizable stages, why is it that exacerbation and escalation can be brought on quickly by social change and uncertainty?

3. *The phenomenon of stabilization.* This point relates to the virtual arrest of deterioration under certain conditions. Kitwood suggests that given an appropriate social, relational, and spiritual environment, a degree of "rementing" can take place. Andrew Sixsmith and colleagues, who undertook a study of "homely homes" where the care was of quite a high quality. They found clear examples of rementing or measurable recovery of powers that apparently had been lost; a degree of cognitive decline often ensued, but it was far slower than that which had been typically expected when people with dementia are in long term care."[369] This process of rementing is recognized within the literature but remains under research.[370] This is not to claim that dementia can somehow be cured through relationships, but it suggests that relationships may have a larger role than is generally recognized in the creation and maintenance of the symptoms of dementia.

Kitwood indicates that the standard paradigm is lacking in both conceptual and empirical grounds. A frame work that has greater explanatory power is required; a different story needs to be told. Kitwood points out not that dementia has no neurological basis. Rather than going for a full-blown social constructionist approach, he was criticized for accepting the medical model of dementia.[371] He is comfortable holding on to the types of understanding that frame dementia as a neurological condition that has multiple causes. It is the singularity and directness of the line of causality that is of particular concern for him. The standard paradigm focuses its gaze on such things as neurological damage caused by strokes, Alzheimer's disease, pathogenic genetic configurations, and so forth. In this view, the line of causality is assumed to be quite straightforward: pathology + brain = dementia. Kitwood argues that such linear configurations of causality fail to take into account the relationship of the brain to the mind and the relationships of the mind and brain to society.

In Kitwood's other way of thinking, the mind receiving and processing of experiences it receives from its encounters with society actually impacts the neurology of the brain. Put it differently, the experiences and the relationships that persons have impact deeply the ways in which their brains come to be structured—something that is true for everyone. Kitwood proposes that the particular ways in which people with dementia experience their social worlds, and in particular the negative ways in which they are framed and treated by others, have an impact on the structures of their brains and *cause,* or at least exacerbate, the process of neurological decline, and also shape and form the symptoms that emerge within the lives of people with dementia. If this is the case, then the standard understanding of the direction of the progression from neurological damage to dementia might require an added dimension that acknowledges the impact of the mind on brain and relationships of mind to society.

Examining What It Means to Be "Your-Self"

Sabat has takes up, further developes, and in important ways offer further verification of Kitwood's thinking in three areas

Positioning. This refers to how an observer perceives and responds to a person with dementia. Perception emerges from presumptions and presuppositions, which develop through the various stories that persons learn to tell about the experience of dementia. These are not always the same thing as reality. The key about a presumption is that somehow people with dementia have gone, that they have lost their "self" or "themselves." It means the subjective "self' becomes eroded to such an extent that it eventually disappears due to the person's gradually failing neurology. The matter is whether the self is present or destroyed in dementia.[372] The term "self" generally seems to be about whether or not that which is essential for person to be aware of selfhood still remains in the context of advanced dementia. More philosophically, am "I" still "me" when "I" have forgotten who "I" am? Presumptions about the loss of self are what lie behind a good deal of malicious social psychology and negative social positioning. If one does not believe the person standing there is "really there," in the same way that one assumes oneself to be "really there," then the "there" person is liable to position the "not there" person in categories that are negative, depersonalizing, and inaccurate.

The Inner Self. To explore the nature of the self, it will be good to reflect on precisely what an "inner self" means when they somehow are "gone." Hans Reinder describes the self as "that part of me where I am with myself."[373] This implies that the self is something that is internal, an aspect of who I think I am that only I can access. It is this sense of inner space of "selfness" that has been deeply influential in the history of Western thought. To be myself, I have to be aware of myself, and the place where I find myself is within me, via my inner concept of who I am. It is this subjective sense of inner space, which is "me," that people with dementia are assumed to be losing. To lose myself is to lose that which makes me who I am, that which provides me with my "inner" sense of who I am. If that is so, any implicit or explicit assumptions that the self is destroyed by dementia inevitably will open up the possibility of malicious social psychology and negative positioning. There are, however, good reasons to think that the self is not destroyed by the decline in neurological processes that mark dementia—not least because there are good reasons to believe that the self is not in fact as "inner" as we might assume.[374]

More precisely, people ask what it might mean for the self to be located within their "inside process." Where exactly is the "inside"? The mind, an aspect of who they are that they normally would assume to be inside of them, does in fact have a significant external social component. People's minds are both personal and social. The idea that the "self," whatever that turns out to be, should be defined by that which is "inner" is not a complete description. Wittgenstein drew attention to the fact that human beings experience things prior to naming them and taking them "inward" toward the development of an experience of mind/self.[375] Babies have a variety of primal experiences when they first experience the world, which they express using external behaviors. As they grow up, they are taught to conceptualize these primal experiences by using particular forms of language. Such words and response to them vary across contexts and cultures. In other words, the various languages that children learn while constructing their different "inner" worlds come with a whole series of meanings and connotations linked to traditions and communities. Thus the "inner" is much more "outer" than it first appears to be.

The languages that children learn from those around them thus form the structures of their experience of their "inner life," and experience that they later are taught to name and understand as their "mind" and/ or "sense of self." The nature and meaning of the language children learn provide the conceptual structure and shape of their minds. The apparently "inner" structure of individual minds are actually found to be the product of "outer" experiences that are drawn "inward" and become experiences that later are define as mind. Thus, the "inner" experience of mind turns out to be a thoroughly "outer" reality and social construct.

What is true for the mind is also true for the "self." In what sense can the self be "inner" when most of what persons know about themselves actually emerges from their relational encounters, their outer experience? It is certain the self inevitably is outer and social even if it feels inner. Owen Thomas shows that the sense of interiority—the feeling or belief that the mind and the self are somehow interior to the body and separated from the wider community—is in fact

A spatial metaphor for something that is non-spatial. It is a metaphor; it makes no sense to say that the self, consciousness, mind, or spirit is literally inside the body. But the reference of interiority, while non-spatial, is localized. It is somehow related to the body and not entirely apart from the body, although the theological and philosophical traditions are divided on this issue.[376]

It is at least open to challenge that the idea of the mind being individual and separated from other minds and selves is something that is only "inner." The mind and the self emerge from relationships and are formed and sustained by and in relationships.[377] That being so, neurological damage may alter certain perceptions (in self and others) of a person's "inner self," but it does not destroy the self, as the self always belongs to a broader community.

A Social Model of the Self. Seeing the "inner self" as definitive of the nature of the self serves as background for understanding the way in which Sabat's idea about excess disability and malicious social positioning fit in with his broader agenda, which is to show that people with dementia do not experience a loss of self. Sabat advocates strongly that dementia does not destroy a person's sense of self. The self can be sustained through appropriate relational encounters. Sabat indicates from quantitative research on people with dementia, including those in the advanced stages, that the self remains intact and can be encountered if caregivers can find the means and the insight to see it and to recognize its presence and stay with it effectively.

Sabat's model of self is quite different from others. For him, the self is something that is constructed within the relational dialectic that goes on between individuals and their communities.

APPENDIX E

Alzheimer's Disease in Chinese Culture and Tradition

China has become an aging society in the past 20 years. As a result, no healthcare problem looms larger in China than Alzheimer's disease, the most common cause of dementia and the most common neurodegenerative disease. It is the fastest growing major disease on the mainland, diagnosed for at least 9.5 million among people age greater than 65 years old and perhaps as many undiagnosed cases. Thus, the higher mortality rates and lower life expectancies are seen in Alzheimer's disease patients relative to the general Chinese population. The annual cost per patient was $19,144 and total annual costs were $167.74 billion in 2015. It is predicted to reach $507.49 billion in 2030 and $1.489 trillion in 2050.[378]

Essay: Alzheimer's Just Killed My Dad and the Chinese Shame is Finally Over by Ray Kwong[379]

Many immigrants—even after decades in the U.S.—hang onto the view that dementia, of which 72 to 80% is caused by Alzheimer's, is part of normal aging. While there is no doubt that Alzheimer's disease is a horrible affliction for anyone who gets it and those it afflicts in turn, when you are of Chinese descent, or other East Asian shame-based lineage, the extra cultural baggage makes life a living hell. Here is a sampling of some of the punishment that Ray had to deal with:

- No one, not even aunt #7, ever thought Dad had Alzheimer's.
- My Mom said "kill me now" every time I brought up assisted living.
- The word "yes" took on a new meaning ("no," go away).
- Attaining harmony meant not having talks cranked up to 11.
- The loss of "face" became a threat more serious than meals without rice.
- Being the #1 son was no longer a perk.
- My dad did not fight for the bill anymore at dim sum.
- He also suddenly thought Panda Express was authentic.

Granted, Chinese are not all alike. But many immigrants—even after decades in the U.S.—hang onto the predominant Chinese view that dementia is part of the normal aging process. Worse, they literally call dementia—which is not itself a disease but instead a wide range of symptoms that reduce a person's ability to perform everyday activities—"old age, dull-witted disease."

Ray Kwong and His Father, Benny Kwong with Dementia's

"To this day, most Chinese people don't even know Alzheimer's is a disease," said Dr. Gerald T. Lim, assistant professor of neurology at the USC Alzheimer's Disease Research Center, of perceptions in China, where more than 9.5 million are afflicted by the disease and as many as 90 percent of cases go undiagnosed.

As astounding as that sounds, it is even more appalling when you consider that as many as one out of every five Alzheimer's patients worldwide is Chinese, according to Alzheimer's Disease International's latest World Alzheimer Report. For the majority of Chinese, it is simple. "When an older person starts to lose his memory, the people around him say it's just part of getting old, no one can escape it and that everyone will be like this eventually," Lim said. "To this day, most Chinese people don't even know Alzheimer's is a disease." The misconceptions are not surprising. There are fewer than 300 doctors in China qualified to diagnose and treat Alzheimer's, and only four hospitals specializing in dementia, according to a report in *The Lancet Medical Journal* in 2013.

With awareness levels so low and the Confucian concept of "filial piety" so strong, caring for dementia sufferers in China falls on family members with little or no support from the state. "It is assumed that families will take care of these things, and family members, in turn, feel they should be able to handle it by themselves," said Eric Miller from Virginia Tech, an expert on aging and intergenerational relationships in China.

Born Identity

In July 1941, Kwong Fook Mah, 17, set foot alone on the docks of the Port of Los Angeles after a three-week voyage from Hong Kong aboard the SS President Coolidge. His parents, having fled to Macau from Japanese-occupied Zhongshan, had planned to send him and his four siblings one at a time to the safety of America, a world away from the escalating conflict between China and Japan and an ongoing Chinese civil war that had no end in sight. But when the U.S. entered the fray of World War II later that year, the plan was trashed. Young Kwong, the first to make the journey, never saw his parents, sisters, or brothers again. Distant relatives in Chinatown took him in, he enrolled in high school, worked as a busboy, and adopted an English name from one of the most popular celebrities of a war-torn decade, radio star Jack Benny.

With the U.S. becoming a major ally of China against Japan, Benny tried to enlist in the army, spending seven months at Camp Howze, an infantry training center located in Gainesville, Texas, before doctors sent him home for having flat feet. Long before Alzheimer's robbed him of his understanding of visual images and spatial relationships, Benny was adept at ignoring visual images and spatial relationships. Disappointed but not discouraged, he moved on, went to college, and in 1951, landed a job at a major aerospace and defense contracting company, where for the next 40 years he worked on teams that engineered everything from the first U.S. soft landing on the moon and ion propulsion engines to night-fighting attack helicopters and laser-guided weapons systems now in service with over 45 militaries.

As recently as Father's Day, the day before my dad passed away as I write this, my dad Benny could vividly describe nearly every detail of trips he took as a young boy to Shanghai to visit his father, who worked in the city as a trader. He just could not remember what he had for breakfast—or much of anything else—and if not for oral histories and a lot of legwork, his immigrant story would be lost. He had Alzheimer's disease, a terrifying, degenerative brain disorder afflicting an estimated 5.4 million Americans. The malady slowly destroys memory and thinking skills, and eventually the ability to carry out the simplest tasks. Recent estimates say it is the third leading cause of death in the U.S., just behind heart disease and cancer.

Feel the Burn

Denial is a common thing for everyone when it comes to the early stages of Alzheimer's, but the Chinese seem to take it to the nth degree, creating a barrier to timely diagnosis tougher to scale than the Great Wall of China. His mother, for example, infuriatingly refused to accept or even acknowledge that my dad had Alzheimer's, responding to every attempt to tell her otherwise with the evil eye and a terse reply of: "He's fine." *This, while he asked her the same question over and over like a broken record, "read" the newspaper upside down and couldn't even recognize himself in family photos.* Older relatives were not much help either. "I just saw your dad and he's eating," was a comment I often got, as if eating makes everything all right (it's a Chinese thing.) *This, while my dad had no clue what day it was, and was deathly afraid that someone would steal his underwear.*

Friends of his generation, while well meaning, were also useless. "He doesn't look like he has Alzheimer's," they would say—never mind that you cannot tell whether someone has Alzheimer's just by looking. *This, while my dad struggled to recall their names, could not order from a menu and had trouble walking ten feet without bumping into something.* Meanwhile, my dad insisted he was fine. *This, while he did not know how old he was,*

could not remember his grandkids' names and sometimes forgot to breathe.
It turns out there is a reason for this madness. Not a good one, but better
than none at all.

A Great Leap Backwards

As naive and primitive as it may seem, most Chinese Americans try
to deal with their mental health issues as if they lived in the ancestral
homeland—without outside help, even from doctors—for fear of the
shame, guilt, and stigma that this knowledge might bring upon the family,
according to the late Evelyn Lee, author of *Working with Asian Americans:
a Guide for Clinicians.* She quotes Lim from USC:

> It's this skewed view based on the cultural beliefs of
> Chinese families within two or three generations of
> immigration to the United States that often delays
> diagnosis of neuro-degenerative diseases like Alzheimer's,
> amyotrophic lateral sclerosis, and Parkinson's, as well as
> treatable mental illnesses like anxiety, depression, and
> schizophrenia.

In my dad's case, my mother's unflinching refusal to acknowledge
that something was horribly wrong with him and her shame-driven
obsession to keep his condition under the radar not only delayed my
dad's diagnosis, but also delayed proper care and management of the
disease for almost two years. While drugs cannot cure Alzheimer's or
stop its progression, they could have slowed his cognitive decline and
helped manage memory loss, thinking and reasoning problems, and day-
to-day function.

Do Not Make My Mistake

My bad for not taking things into my own hands sooner, but you do not
have to make the same mistake. Do yourself a favor and make a point to

recognize the early signs and symptoms of Alzheimer's, and take your loved one to the doctor if you notice *any* of them.

Do not let older family members stop you from doing the right thing. Their fear of public humiliation and scorn—even the notion that Alzheimer's or any mental illness reflects poorly on family lineage—is total bulls—t. You turned out OK, am I right? Do not cave-in. You will save yourself a lot of stress, frustration, sleepless nights, and anxiety about the future. For Chinese families, Alzheimer's presents unique cultural challenges. Research shows that duty to parents and use of herbal medicine influence cultural responses to the disease. Complex cultural issues often affect the care of Chinese people who have Alzheimer's disease.[380]

If dementia were a country, its economy would rank eighteenth, between Turkey and Indonesia. The total estimated global cost of dementia in 2010 was slated to be $604 billion, according to Alzheimer's Disease International. In 2020, Alzheimer's and other dementias will cost just the U.S. $305 billion, including $206 billion in Medicare and Medicaid payments. Unless a treatment to slow, stop or prevent the disease is developed, in 2050, Alzheimer's is projected to cost globally more than $1.1 trillion. The total number of people with dementia is projected to reach 82 million in 2030 and 152 million in 2050. Much of this increase is attributable to the rising numbers of people with dementia living in low- and middle-income countries. The sharpest increase in the 35.6 million people across the world with dementia is now occurring in rapidly developing regions, especially in China.

Yu-Ping Chang, a University at Buffalo[381] assistant professor of nursing, published a study in *Perspectives in Psychiatric Care* on the unique challenges experienced by Chinese families in Taiwan when confronting Alzheimer's. She also received a grant from the Alzheimer's Association to explore how Chinese immigrant families in San Francisco cope with Alzheimer's disease and how they use traditional Chinese herbal medicines to treat it. Fundamental to Chang's research is the Chinese concept of filial piety or "Xiào," which is inherited from the Confucian ideals and requires children from birth to death to be respectful of parents and ancestors.

The article finds that the Taiwanese stories differ from their mainland Chinese and Hong Kong counterparts in three ways: First, the onset of dementia is largely an unforeseen calamity for the Taiwanese storytellers, while it is an anticipatable life circumstance for the mainland Chinese and Hong Kong storytellers. Second, the Taiwanese storytellers tend to locate the cause for the deterioration of their elderly family member in illness, while the mainland Chinese and Hong Kong storytellers tend to explain away the deterioration of their elderly family member as normative aging. Third, the Taiwanese storytellers maintain their existing identities when faced with the newfound challenge of family caregiving in dementia, while the mainland Chinese and Hong Kong storytellers commonly appropriate the former culturally embodied identity of the family member whom they now care for.

Grown children practicing Chinese filial piety, Chang notes, are expected to reciprocate their parents' love for them with respect and gratitude. When parents become ill, the children are to be solely and directly responsible for their care. Until recently, this did not include placing parents under the care of others. For her study, "Decision-Making Processes of Nursing Home Placement among Chinese Family Caregivers," she traveled to Taiwan to interview the caregivers of parents with Alzheimer's disease and found that the chief concern for them was the conflict between the need to place a loved one in a nursing home and filial piety.

Caring for parents with Alzheimer's disease presents many of the same challenges to modern Chinese children as it does children in the U.S. Caregivers often experience each day as having thirty-six hours. Even when one or more children can be at home with a parent, parents with dementia often become too difficult to care for, placing the burden on the children to find institutional means of care. Among the Chinese, however, not living up to the ideals of filial piety can result in feelings of deep shame and failure far beyond the guilt that Western caregivers experience when they have to make the decision to place a parent or elder in a nursing home. Following are factors involved in the decision:

- Initiating the placement decision—prompted by deteriorating dementia behaviors
- Assessing and weighing the decision—information gathering and involvement of the entire family
- Finalizing the decision—family consensus was essential
- Evaluating the decision—reconciling tense family relationships, examining quality of care

Though the demands of filial piety weighed heavily on caregivers during each phase, Chang found that they could compensate for it by finding the best nursing home, gaining the consensus of the entire family about placement (even aunts and uncles), visiting the nursing home frequently, and checking in with the parent often to ensure ongoing quality of care.

For her two-year research project funded by the Alzheimer's Association in 2009, Chang studied the relationship between Chinese immigrants' cultural beliefs and medication use in the San Francisco Bay area. Many Chinese immigrants self-medicate using traditional Chinese herbal medicine (TCHM), in addition to their regularly prescribed medications, without telling their physicians, Chang says. Or, perhaps, their Western physicians never asked them about the use of TCHM due to a lack of awareness of the cultural issues.

As part of this study, Chang spent time with Alzheimer's disease sufferer, Sir Charles K. Kao, 2009 Nobel Prize winner in physics (known as the father of broadband) and his wife, Gwen. Charles was diagnosed with Alzheimer's at about the same time he and his wife were notified about the Nobel Prize. Afterward, Gwen became an advocate for Alzheimer's funding in California. According to her, the use of TCHM is common in this population, and many Chinese Americans suffering with Alzheimer's feel shame and, thus, do not seek help from medical professionals. Because of the complexity of such cultural and medical issues, Chang's research targeted family caregivers. She noted that patients suffering from dementia are often poor historians and could not accurately describe their medication use. Thus, many Chinese-American children caring for a parent may dutifully continue to give TCHM out of filial piety.

"I think Chinese-Americans have different perspectives regarding dementia, such as attributing it to normal aging, the yin-yang imbalance, mental illness, fate, and the sins of their ancestors," Chang wrote. "These may potentially influence the way they take care of their loved ones. Thus, I want to understand if Chinese-American family caregivers use TCHM to treat dementia-related symptoms and how their cultural beliefs and other factors influence their medication."

The study aimed to determine the scope of TCHM use, the common ingredients selected, and the patterns of patient-clinician communication regarding TCHM use. Eventually, Chang plans to design culturally appropriate interventions for Chinese American family caregivers to better manage their caregiving task as well as maintain their own health. Chang hoped her research would instruct healthcare providers that Chinese families—patients and caregivers—may be at risk because of the cultural stressors involved in making such decisions. She was especially concerned for culturally isolated Chinese immigrant families in the U.S.

For example, in San Francisco, Chang pointed out, nursing homes have large populations of Taiwanese, Mandarin, and Cantonese immigrants where patients and their families have others who speak their language and understand their culture. But in many parts of the world, Chinese residents in nursing homes are alone. "Chinese endure things often without complaint so they will not communicate distress," Chang noted. "Nurses need to be aware of this and other cultural differences so that they can work more effectively with patients and families."

APPENDIX F

Helpful Scriptures

The mind, the will and/or subconscious are stricken. The soul needs to be healed. Scriptures refer to restoring or completing the soul can be effective in combating the disease. We need to **hope** in the Lord, claim his **promises**, express **thanks** for what he has done and **praise** him (Rom. 4:18–21), and pray in expectation that he will hear and answer our prayers (1 John 5:14-15).

- **Hope**:

  Psalms 55:16, "As for me, I will call upon the God and the Lord shall save me."

  Psalms 124:8, "Our help is in the name of Lord who made heaven and the earth."

  Psalms 56:13, "For you have delivered my soul from death; will you not deliver my feet from falling that I may walk before God in the light of the living?"

  Psalms 62:1, "Truly my soul waits upon God; from him comes my salvation."

- **Promises**:

  Psalms 107:6, "Then they cried unto the Lord in their trouble and he delivered them out of their distress."

1 Kings 1:29, "The Lord redeemed my soul out of all distress."

Job 33:28, "God will deliver his soul from going into the pit and his life shall see the light."

Isaiah 54:15, "If anyone does attack you, it will not be my doing, whoever attacks you will surrender to you."

2 Timothy 1:7, "For God has not given us a spirit of fear, but of power, and of love and of sound mind."

- **Thanksgiving**
  Psalms 86:13, "For great is your mercy toward me and you have delivered my soul from the lowest hell *of the disease*."

  Psalms 30:3, "Oh Lord you have brought up my soul from grave. You have kept me alive that I should not go down to the pit."

  Psalms 94:17, "Unless the Lord had been my help. My soul had almost dwelled in silence."

- **Praise**
  Psalms 55:18, "He has delivered my soul in peace from battle *of the disease* that was against me."

  Psalms 103:1–6, "Bless the Lord oh my soul and all is within me bless his holy name. Bless the Lord of my soul . . . who heals all my diseases, who redeems my life from destruction, who crowns me with loving kindness and tender mercy."

There are more encouraging and comfort scriptures readers can search for to suit their needs in specific situations.

END NOTES

Preface

1 Margaret Goodell, "Caring for Those with Dementia: Through Creative Imagine," *Health & Medicine Journal* (July 2013). She is professor and researcher at Baylor College of Medicine.

2 T. R. Elliot, M. Parker, and L. Roff, "Family Caregivers and Health Care Providers: Developing Partnerships for Continuum of Care and Support," in Ronda Talley, *The Multiple Dimensions of Caregiving and Disability* (New York: Springier Press, 2012), 25.

3 Karem Gram, "This is What Love is," in *The Vancouver Sun*, B3 (August 16, 2007).

4 Lisa Genova, *Still Alice* (New York: Simon & Schuster, 2009).

5 Ibid., 192.

6 Oliver Sacks, *The Man who Mistook His Wife for a Hat* (New York: Summit Books, 1985), 1.

7 T. Kitwood and S. Benson, eds., *The New Culture of Dementia Cure* (London: Hawker, 1995); Tom Kitwood, *Dementia Reconsidered: The Person Come First* (Maidenhead, UK: Open University Press, 1997).

8 Brevard S. Childs, *Memory and Tradition in Israel* (London: SCM Press, 1962), 34.

9 Bruce K. Waltke, *An Old Testament Theology* (Grand Rapids: Zondervan, 2007), 225–7.

10 John Calvin, *Commentary on Deuteronomy*, Charles Willian Bingham, ed. (Grand Rapids: Baker, 1974), 398–9.

11 Ibid.

12 Sir John Ecceles, the Nobel neuroscientist, his approach was different from what is explored biblically here. He was defending the canons of science from usurping the reductionistic role of scientism. The argument here instead expands the moral significance of memory and indeed of personhood, which calls for reform in our society.

Introduction

13 A quote from Elisabeth Peterson, *Voice of Alzheimer's: Courage, Humor, Hope, and Love in the Face of Dementia* (Cambridge: Da Capo Press, 2004), 57.

14 John Winston, *Dementia: Living in the Memory of God* (London: SCM Press, 2012), 2.

15 Dietrich Bonhoeffer, *Who Am I?: Poetic Insights on Personal Identity* (Minneapolis: Augsburg Books, 2005), 8–9.

16 Unless otherwise notes, all scripture references will use the New Living Translation (NLT).

17 Recent development in Holland indicate that enabling people with dementia to end their lives may be becoming an accepted practice. See Tony Sheldon, "Euthanasia Endorsed in Dutch Patient with Dementia," *British Medical Journal* 10, no. 319 (July 1999): 75.

18 See "Killing Compassion," in Stanley Hauerwas, *Dispatches from the front: Theological Engagement with the Secular* (Durham, NC: Duke University Press, 1994).

19 Ibid.

20 John Swinton and Stephen Pattison, "Moving Beyond Clarity: Toward a Thin, Vague, and Useful Understanding of Spirituality As It Relates to Healthcare in Nursing Care," *Nursing Philosophy* 11, no. 4 (2010): 226–37. A critique of generic approaches to spirituality.

21 See Joel James Shuman and Keith Meador, *Heal Thyself: Spirituality, Medicine, and the Distortion of Christianity* (New York: Oxford University Press, 2001).

22 H. G. Koenig, D. B. Larson, and M.E. McCullough, *Handbook of Religion and Health* (New York: Oxford University Press, 2001).

23 K. I. Pargament, "The Bitter and the Sweet: An Evaluation of the Costs and Benefits of Religiousness," *Psychological Inquiry* 13 (2002): 168–81.

24 G. Bono and M. E. McCollough, "Positive Responses to Benefit and Harm: Bringing Forgiveness and Gratitude into Cognitive Psychotherapy," *Journal of Cognitive Psychotherapy* 20 (2006): 147–58. For a powerful theological critique of this approach, see L. Gregory Johns, *Embodying Forgiveness: A theological Analysis* (Grand Rapids: Wm. B. Eerdmans, 1995).

25 John Swinton, *From Bedlam to Shalom: Toward a Practical Theology of Human Nature, Interpersonal Relationship, and Mental Health Care* (New York: Peter Lang, 2000).

26 Job 8:28: "and this is what he says to all humanity: 'The fear of the Lord is true wisdom; to forsake evil is real understanding.'"

27 John Howard Yoder, *The Original Revolution* (Scottdale, PA: Herald Press, 1971), 116. John Yoder states, "The distinction between church and the world is not a distinction between nature and grace. It is instead, a distinction that denotes

the basic personal postures of men, some confess and others do not confess that Jesus is Lord. The distinction is not God has imposed upon the world by prior metaphysical definition, nor something Christians have built up around themselves. It is all of that in creation that has taken the freedom not yet to believe."

28 See also Andrew B. Newberg, *The Mystical Mind: Probing the Biology of Religious Experience* (Minneapolis: Fortress Press, 1999). We (humans) are embodied creatures, and that what occurs within the bodies inevitably has theological significance.

29 David Keck, *Forgetting Whose We Are: Alzheimer's Disease and Love of God* (Nashville: Abington Press, 1996), 15.

30 Ibid., 15.

31 John Calvin, *Institutes of the Christian Religion* (Philadelphia: Westminster Press, 1960), 35.

32 Ibid.

33 St. Augustine, *Confessions*, in *The Works of Saint Augustine: A Translation for the 21st Century*, 2nd ed. (New York: New City Press, 2001).

34 Anselm of Canterbury, *Proslogion*, M. J. Charlesworth, trans., in *The Major Works*, Brian Davis and G. R. Evans, eds. (New York: Oxford University Press, 1998).

35 Friedrich Daniel and Ernst Schleiermacher, *The Christian Faith* (London: T&T Clark, 1928), 132.

36 Keck, *Forgetting Whose We Are*, 15.

Chapter One

37 Karl Barth, "Strange-New World in the Bible," from Chapter 2 in Karl Barth and Douglas Horton, *The Word of God and the Word of Man* (Smith Publishers, 1958), 28, Kindle. Barth was a Swiss reformed theologian and pastor.

38 John Swinton and Harriet Mowat, *Practical Theology and Qualitative Research Method* (London: SCM Press, 2006), 6. The term "practices" relates to forms of divinely inspire human action that are rooted in Christian beliefs about the world and the way that God and human beings perceive and act within the world.

39 In James 2:19, the apostle observes that anybody can know things about God. Knowledge *about* God is useless without knowledge *of* God. To know God is something quite different from knowing about God.

40 Walter Brueggemann, *Redescribing Reality: What We Do When We Read the Bible* (London: SCM Press, 2009).

41 Neil MacDonald, *Karl Barth and the Strange New World within the Bible: Barth, Wittgenstein, and the Metadilemmas of the Enlightenment* (Cumbria: Paternoster Press, 2006).

42 "I tell you the truth . . . a plentiful harvest of new lives" (John 12:24).

43 "But he said to me, 'My grace is sufficient for you' . . . so that Christ's power may rest on me" (2 Corinthians 12:9, NIV).

44 "Take my yoke upon you . . . and you will find rest for your souls" (Matthew 11:29, NIV). The statement, "I am humble and gentle at heart is profound. Jesus, who is God, claims that his very essence he is humble and gentle. Somewhere within the heart of God, humility and gentleness reign. To be humble and gentle is to be like God.

45 "For the wisdom of this world is foolish to God. As the Scriptures say, 'He traps the wise in the snare of their own cleverness'" (1 Corinthians 3:19).

46 Brueggemann, Redescribing Reality, 38.

47 Walter Brueggemann, The Word that Redescribes the World: The Bible and Discipleship (Minneapolis: Augsburg Fortress Press, 2006), 49.

48 "God saw all that he has made . . . and there was morning—the sixth day" (Genesis 1:31).

49 "For God so love the world, that whoever believes in him shall not perish but have eternal life" (John 3:16, NIV).

50 "'For I know the plans I have for you . . . Plans to give you hope and a future'" (Jeremiah 29:11, NIV).

51 Walter Brueggemann, "Cadences which Redescribe: Speech among Exiles," Journal for Preachers 27, no. 3 (Easter 1994): 10–17.

52 Hilde Lindemann Nelson, Damaged Identities, Narrative Repair (New York: Cornel University Press, 2001), especially Chapters 3, 4.

53 People with dementia are not capable human beings. Incapable means an all-inclusive adjective.

54 Christine Borden, Who Will I Be When I Die? (Melbourne: Harper Collins, 1998). Diagnosed at forty-six with dementia, her book details the beginning of her illness.

55 Matthew 16:13–16, NIV. The key thing for Jesus here, in the midst of a confusing narrative, is that Peter alone noticed who Jesus really was and bore witness to the fact that he was Messiah, Son of living God. There is a powerful principle here for dementia care.

56 Karl Barth, Church Dogmatics, 4 vols., Thomas F. Torrance, ed., Geoffrey W. Bromiley, trans. (New York: T & T Clark, 2009), I–179.

57 Elie Wiesel, Inside a Library and The Stranger in Bible (New York: Hebrew Union College, Jewish institute of Religion, 1981), 28.

58 Jonathan Cohen, in Encounter with Mystery, Frances Young, ed. (London: Darton, Longman & Todd, 1997), 29.

59 Ibid., 157.

60 Michael Ignatieff, Scare Tissue (London: Penguin Books, 1993).

Chapter 2

61 Steven R. Sabat, *The Experience of Alzheimer's Disease: Life through a Tangled Veil* (Oxford: Blackwell, 2001), 4.

62 Richard Cheston and Michael Bender, *Understanding Dementia: The Man with the Worried Eyes* (London: Jessica Kinsley Publishers, 1999), 53.

63 Gloria J. Sterin, "Essay on a Word: A Lived Experience of Alzheimer's Disease," *Dementia* (February 2002): 1.

64 Broxmeyer's paper can be found in *Medical Hypotheses* 64, no. 4 (2005): 699–705.

65 The *Diagnostic and Statistical Manual of Mental Health Disorders* (DSM), currently in the 5th edition, is the primary diagnostic publication by which psychiatrists and psychologists make diagnoses. Produced by the American Psychiatric Association (APA) and others, it classifies categories and criteria of mental health disorders for both adults and children.

66 Wolfgang Kohlor, *Gestalt Psychology* (New York: Horace Liveright, 1929), 250. He anticipates Wittingenstein's later aphorism, "The human body is the best picture of the human soul." See Ludwig Wittgenstein, *Philosophical Investigations*, G. E. M. Anscombe, trans. (New York: Boni & Liveright Publishing, 1933), 178.

67 Ian Hacking, "Autistic Autobiography," Philosophical Transactions of the Royal Society B (May 27, 2009), 1467–73.

68 Steve R. Sabat and Rom Harré, "The Alzheimer's Disease Sufferer as a Semiotic Subject," *Philosophy, Psychiatry, Psychology* 1 (1994):145–60. For an extended empirical development of this point, see Sabat, *The Experiment of Alzheimer's Disease.*

69 Jaber F. Gubrium, "The Social Preservation of Mind: The Alzheimer's Disease Experience," *Symbolic Interaction* 9, no. 1 (Spring 1986): 37–51.

70 Robert Bogdan and Steven J, Taylor, "Relationship with Severely Disabled People: The Social Construction of Humanness," *Social Problems* 36, no. 2 (April 1989).

71 This point gain further poignancy in the light of discussion of the social construction of thinking. See David Keck, *Forgetting Whose We Are: Alzheimer's Disease and the Love of God* (Nashville: Abingdon Press, 1996)

72 Ludwig Wittgenstein, *Philosophical Investigations*, 4th ed., E. M. Anscombe, P. M. S. Hacker, and Joachim Schulte, trans. (Oxford: Wiley Blackwell, 2009).

73 David G. Stern, *Wittgenstein on Mind and Language* (London: Oxford University Press, 1985).

Chapter 3

74 Martin Niemöller was a German born theologian, poet, author, and Lutheran pastor. This is his one of 25 famous quotes in poetic form, written in the mid-1950s. See http://www.azquotes.com/author 20566-martin-niemöller.

75 On the linguistic "killing" of people with dementia, see Tom Kitwood, "Toward the Reconstruction of an Organic Mental Disorder," in Alan Radley, ed., *Worlds of Illness: Biographical and Cultural Perspectives on Health and Disease* (London: Routledge, 1995).

76 John Locke, *An Essay Concerning Human Understanding*, Peter H. Nidditch, ed. (Oxford: Clarendon Press, 1975), E II, xxvii, 335.

77 Peter Singer, *Practical Ethics* (Cambridge: Cambridge University Press, 1979), particularly Chapter 7, "Taking Life Humans." For a full-blown Christian critique of Singer's ethics, see Gordon R. Preece, *Rethinking Peter Singer: A Christian Critique* (Downers Grove: InterVarsity Press, 2002).

78 Ibid., 83.

79 Peter Singer, *Rethinking Life and Death* (New York: St. Martin's Press, 1995), 197–8.

80 John Wyatt, "What Is a Person?" *Nucleus* (January 2004): 10–15; quotation on 10. For a more fully developed argument, see John Wyatt, *Matter of Life and Dead: Human Dementia in the Life of the Christian Faith* (Nottingham: InterVarsity Press, 2009), 44–6.

81 Ibid., 47.

82 Tom Kitwood, *Dementia Reconsidered: The Person Comes First* (Buckingham: Open University Press, 1997), 9.

83 Eva Kittay, *Love's Labor: Essay on Women, Equality, and Dependency* (New York: Routledge, 1999), 2–4.

84 Michael Specter, "The Dangerous Philosopher," *The New Yorker* 6 (September 1999): 55.

85 Ibid.

86 Ibid.

87 Ibid.

88 Ibid.

89 Peter Singer, *Practical Ethics*, 3rd ed. (Cambridge: Cambridge University Press, 2011).

90 Carl Sandburg was a Swedish American poet, journalist, and biographer. This quote may be in one of his poem collections published in 1918. See http://www.brainy quote.com/quote/carl_sandburg_345254.

91 David Edvardsson, Winblad Bengt, and P. O. Sandman, "Person-Centered Care of People with Severe Alzheimer's Disease: Status and Ways Forward," *The Lancet: Neurology* 7, no.4 (April 2008): 362–7; quotation on 363.

92 Ibid.

93 N. Mead and P. Bower, "Patient-Centeredness: A Conceptual Framework and Review of the Empirical Literature," *Social Science and Medicine* 51 (2000): 1087–110.

94 B. McCormack, "Person-Centeredness in Gerontological Nursing: An Overview of the Literature," *International Journal of Older People Nursing* 13 (2004): 31–8.

95 A. Titchen, "Skilled Companionship in Professional Practice," *in Practice Knowledge and Expertise in the Health Professions*, J. Higgs and A. Titchen, eds. (Oxford: Butterworth-Heinemann, 2001).

96 M. R. Nolan, S. Davies, J. Brown, J. Keady, and J. Nolan, "Beyond 'Person-Centered' Care: A New Vision for Gerontological Nursing," *Journal of Clinical Nursing* 13 (2004): 45–53.

97 T. Packer, "Turning Rhetoric into Reality: Person-Centered Approaches for Community Mental Health Nursing," *in Community Mental Health Nursing and Dementia Care*, J. Keady, C. Clarke, and T. Adams, eds. (Maidenhead: Open University Press, 2003), 104–19.

98 Edvardsson, et al., "Person-Centered Care of People with Severe Alzheimer's Disease," 363.

99 See *Spirituality and Personhood in Dementia*, Albert Jewell, ed. (London: Jessica Kingsley Publishers, 2011).

100 Tom Kitwood, "The Experience of Dementia," *Aging and Metal Health* 1, no. 1 (1997): 13–22; quotation on 16.

101 Cultures that contain the type of malignant social psychology explored here are deeply implicated in the formation and sustaining of the perception and experiences of dementia.

102 Tom Kitwood, *Dementia Reconsidered: The Person Comes First* (Buckingham: Open University Press, 1997), 8.

103 Martin Buber, *I and Thou* (Edinburgh: T&T Clark, 1958).

104 Molly C. Haslam, *A Constructive Theology of Intellectual Disability: Human Being as Mutuality and Response* (New York: Fordham University Press, 2012), 68.

105 Ibid.

106 Kitwood, *Dementia Reconsidered*, 10-11.

107 Jan Dewing, "Personhood and Dementia: Revisiting Tom Kitwood's Ideas," *International Journal of older People Nursing* 3 (March 2008): 3–13; quotation on 10.

108 Stuart Charmé, "The Two I-Thou Relations in Martin Buber's Philosophy," *Harvard Theological Review* 70, no. 12 (January–April 1977): 161–75: quotation on 162.

109 Buber, *I and Thou*, 136.

110 Ibid.

111 Haslam, *A Constructive Theology of Intellectual Disability*, 69.

Chapter 4

112 Jean Vanier, a Switzerland-born Canadian Catholic philosopher and theologian, founder of L'Arche (1964) and Faith and Light (1971) in France. *Befriending the Stranger* (Mahwah, NJ: Paulist Press, 2010).

113 Robert Spaemann, *Persons: The Difference between "Someone" and "Something,"* trans. Oliver O'Donovan (Oxford: Oxford University Press, 2006), 257.

114 Ibid.

115 Ibid., 253.

116 Ibid., 255–6.

117 Berndt Wannenwetsch, "Angels with Clipped Wings: The Disabled as Key to the Recognition of Personhood," in John Swinton and Brian Brok, eds., *Theology, Disability, and the New Genetics: Why Science Needs the Church* (London: T&T Clark, 2007), 187.

118 Ibid.

119 Jurgen Moltmann, *The Trinity and the Kingdom of God: The Doctrine of God* (London: SCM Press Ltd., 1993), 17; *God in Creation: An Ecological Doctrine of Creation* (London: SCM Press Ltd., 1985).

120 John Zizioulas, *Being in Communion* (Crestwood, NY: St. Vladimirs Seminary Press, 1985); Christoph Schwobel and Colin Gunton, eds., *Persons: Divine and Human* (Edinburgh: T & T Clark, 1991).

121 Karen Kilby, "Perichoresis and Projection: Problem with Social Doctrine of Trinity," *New Blackfriars* 81, no. 956 (2000): 432–45. Peter Kevern, "What Sort of a God is to be Found in Dementia?: A Survey of Theological Responses and an Agenda for Their Development," *Theology* 113, no. 873 (May 2010): 174–82.

122 Biblical creationism is an intentionally specific term; otherwise, it would be just another "theistic science," also called "theistic evolution" or "evolutionary creation," which can differ widely from biblical creationism. See the movie, *Is Genesis History?* The free e-book, *Why Sex Is the Best Argument for Creation*, has more detail. Download here: https://isgenesishistory.com/free-ebook/.

123 Walter Brueggemann, *An Unsettling God: The Heart of Hebrew Bible* (Minneapolis: Fortress Press, 2009), 60.

124 Ibid.

125 St. Augustine, quoted in Gilbert Meilaender, "*Terra es Animata*: On Having a Life," *The Hasting Center Report* 23, no. 4 (July–August 1993): 25–32; quotation on 25.

126 Wendell Berry, *The Art of the Commonplace: The Agrarian Essay of Wendell Berry* (Berkeley: Counter Point Press, 2002), 313.

127 Glenn E. Whitlock, "The Structure of Personality in Hebrew Psychology," *Interpretation: A Journal of Bible and Theology* 14, no. 1 (January 1960): 3–14; quotations on 8–9.

128 Ray S. Anderson, *On Being Human: Essay in Theological Anthropology* (Grand Rapids: Wm. B. Eerdmanns, 1982), 5.

129 Walter Brueggemann points out, "The articulation of 'breathed out dust' in order to become a 'living being' precludes any dualism. It is unfortunate that 'living being' (Nephesh) is commonly rendered 'soul,' which in classical thought has made a contrast to the 'body,' a distinction precluded in Israel's way of speaking.

Thus the human person is a dependent, vitality-given unity, for which the term *psychosomatic entity* might be appropriate, if that phrasing did not itself reflect a legacy of dualism." See Brueggmann, *An Unsettling God*, 60.

130 John A. T. Robinson, *The Body: A Study in Pauline Theology* (Chicago: Alec R. Allenson, 1952), 14. The Quotation is from J. Pedersen, *Israel: Its Life and Culture*, 2 vols. (London: Oxford University Press, 1963), 171.

131 Glenn Weaver, "Senile Dementia and a Resurrection Theology," *Theology Today* 42 (1986): 444–56: quotation on 446.

132 Berry, *The Art of the Commonplace*, 308.

133 Ibid.

134 "In him was life, and the life was the light of all people" (John 1:4, NRSV).

135 Anderson, *On Being Human*, 21.

136 Naming Adam is the work and desire of God.

137 Adam found his fulfillment, as opposed to his identity, as a human being. Adam was already affirmed as fully human by God's initial entering into a personal relationship with him.

138 The intimate relationship of Adam and Even is not the only type of relationship necessary for fulfilled human existence. The relationship implicit within the Genesis account suggests that human beings are fundamentally relational beings who require relationships at a number of levels for the fulfillment of their temporal existence. This desire to relate is a direct consequence of their being made in the image of a God who desires to relate to them.

139 Josef Pieper, *Faith, Hope, Love* (San Francisco: Ignatius Press, 1997), 164.

140 Ibid.

141 "Then God looked over all he had made, and he saw that it was very good! And evening passed and morning came, marking the sixth day" (Genesis 1:31).

142 Anastasia Scrutton, *Thinking Through Feeling: God, Emotion, Passibility* (New York: Bloombury Academic, 2013), 145. Scrutton is a Frederick J. Crosson Research Fellow at the Center for Philosophy of Religion, University of Notre Dame, USA.

143 See Thomas Aquinas, *Summa Theologica* (Raleigh, NC: Hayes Barton Press, 1925), 899.

144 Berphysiory, *The Art of the Commonplace*, 397.

Chapter 5

145 M. Dean, "Grey Growth," *Lancet* 335 (1990): 1330–1.

146 E. Jamison, *World Population Profile: U.S. Bureau of the Census*, report WP/91 (Washington, DC: U.S. Government Printing Office, 1991).

147 National Institute of Health, "Diagnosis and Treatment of Depression in Late Life," *Consensus Development Conference Statement* 9, no. 3 (1991).

148 J. M. Guralnik, A. Z. LaCroix, D. F. Everett, and M. G. Kovar, "Aging in Eighties: The Prevalence of Comorbidity and its Association with Disability," *Advance Data*, Vital and Health Statistics of National Center of Health Statistics, no. 170 (1992): 1–8.

149 "Demography of Aging," in R. Binstock and L. George, eds., *Handbook of Aging and the Social Sciences*, 3rd ed. (San Diego: Academic Press, 1990), 19–44.

150 Harold G. Koenig and Andrew J. Weaver, *Pastoral Care of Older Adults: Creative Pastoral Care and Counseling Series* (Minneapolis: Fortress Press, 1998), 3.

151 Richard H. Gentzler, Jr., *Aging and Ministry In the 21st Century: An Inquiry Approach* (Nashville: Discipleship Resources, 1989), 29–32.

152 Koenig and Weaver, *Pastoral Care of Older Adults*, 3-4.

153 Kitwood, *Dementia Reconsidered: The Person Comes First* (Buckingham: Open University Press, 1997), 18.

154 John C. Eccles, *Evolution of the Brain: Creation of self* (London: Routledge, 1991), 221–2. Eccles is using Karl Popper's representational model of human neurological evolution, in which the human brain evolves in three stages or World 1, 2, and 3. World 3 is the world of knowledge in the objective sense—i.e., the whole manmade world of culture, including language. It is in the interplay between World 2 and World 1 that a person develops a sense of self and a conscious place in the universe.

155 Kitwood, *Dementia Reconsidered*, 19.

156 Ibid., 17.

157 Clive Baldwin and Andrea Capstick, *Tom Kitwood on Dementia* (Maidenhead: Open University Press, 2007), 77.

158 A good example of this is found in what has come to be known as, "The Nun Study." See Kathryn P. Riley, et al., "Early Life Linguistic Ability, Late Life Cognitive Function, and Neuropathology: Finding from the Nun Study," *Neurobiology of Aging* 26, no. 3 (2005): 341–7.

159 See Murray Lloyd, "Resilience Promotion and its Relevance to the Personhood, Needs of People with Dementia and Other Brain Damage," in Albert Jewell, *Spirituality and Personhood in Dementia* (London: Jessica Kinsley Publishers, 2011), 142–53.

160 Malcolm Jeeves, ed., *From Cells to Souls and Beyond: Changing Portraits of Human Nature* (Grand Rapids: Wm. B. Eerdmans, 2004).

161 Robert Davis, *My Journey into Alzheimer's Disease: Helpful Insights for Family and Friends* (Carol Stream, IL: Tyndale House Publishers, 1989), 53.

162 Ray Anderson, in Warren S. Brown, Nancey Murphy, and H. Newton Malony, eds., *Whatever Happened to the Soul? Scientific and Theological Portraits of Human Nature* (Minneapolis: Fortress Press, 1998), 188.

163 Based on Romans 8:27, NIV.

164 Anderson, in Brown, et al., *Whatever Happened to the Soul?* 188.

165 Nancy Murphy, *Bodies and Souls, or Spirited Bodies?* (Cambridge University Press, 2006), Chapter 1. Also Matthew 10:28 (NIV).

166 Anderson, in Brown, et al., *Whatever Happened to the Soul?* 189.

167 Regan Sutterfield, *Wendell Berry and the Given Life* (Cincinnati: Franciscan Media, 2017), 45. Wendell Berry was a novelist, poet, and essayist, has won many awards, is recognized in the Hall of Fame, and he was a farmer.

168 Iozzio, "The Writing on the Wall," 50.

Chapter 6

169 Arthur Kleinman, *Caregiving: The Soul of Care* (London: Penguin Random House, 2020), 15.

170 American Psychiatric Association, 2000.

171 NLM, Apr. 2017. Childhood dementia is a mental disorder. This condition cannot be categorized as a specific disease, but manifests in the form of various symptoms. If diagnosed, a child will experience quick and progressive mental and physical deterioration over the course of several years—similar to Alzheimer's disease, hence its nickname of "childhood Alzheimer's." Like Alzheimer's, or Niemann-Pick disease type C it has *no cure* and typically leads to death.

172 Lisa Genova, *Still Alice* (New York: Simon & Schuster, 2009).

173 Stanley Jacobson and Elliot M. Marcus, "Higher Cortical Functions," *Neuroanatomy for the Neuroscientist* (January 2008): 375–95.

174 "Behavioural and Neuroimaging Changes after Naming Therapy for Semantic Variable Primary Progressive Aphasia," Neuropsychologia 89 (Aug. 1, 2016): 191–216, accessed Feb. 25, 2021, https://www.sciencedirect.com/science/article/pii/S0028393216302081. From the article: The semantic variant of primary progressive aphasia (svPPA), also known as semantic dementia or fluent PPA, is associated with impaired understanding of word meaning and/or object identity (Patterson et al., 1994, Patterson and Hodges, 1992, Hodges et al., 1992; Hodges, 1999). As a result of semantic loss in SVPPA, the accompanying language ... semantic dementia, also known as semantic variant primary progressive aphasia, is generally considered to be one of three subtypes of primary progressive aphasia, along with progressive non-fluent aphasia and logopaenic dementia.

Chapter 7

175 Michael Ignatieff, *Scare Tissue* (London: Penguin Books, 1993).

176 *The ICD-10 Classification of Mental and Behavioral Disorders: Descriptions and Diagnostic Guideline* (Geneva: WHO, 1992). The ICD is the international standard diagnostic classification resource for all general, epidemiological, and many health management purposes and clinical use. See http://www.who.int/classifications/icd/en/.

177 DSM-5 is the main diagnostic manual used by psychiatrists to make diagnoses. It is produced by the American Psychiatric Association and covers all categories of mental health disorders for both adults and children.

178 Richard Cheston and Michael Bender, *Understanding Dementia: The Man with the Worried Eyes* (London: Jessica Kinsley Publishers, 1999), 51.

179 Warren Kinghorn, "Ordering Mental Disorder: Theology and the Disputed Boundaries of Psychiatric Diagnosis." Unpublished paper presented at the Society of Spirituality, Theology, and Health, 3rd Annual Meeting, Durham, NC, June 17, 2010. See also Warren Kinghorn, "Whose Disorder?: A Constructive MacIntyrean Critic of Psychiatric Nosology," *Journal of Medicine and philosophy Advance* (February 28, 2011): 1–19.

180 Ethan Watters, *Crazy Like Us: The Globalization of the American Psych* (New York: Free Press, 2010).

181 Cheston and Bender, *Understanding Dementia*, 50–1.

182 Ibid., 51. See also Daniel George, *The Myth Of Alzheimer's: What You Aren't Being Told about Today's Most Dreaded Diagnosis* (New York: St. Martin's Press, 2008).

183 Barbara Tuchman, *A Distance Mirror: Calamitous Fourteen Century* (Harmonsworth, UK: Penguin, 1979).

184 Ronald L. Numbers and Ronald C. Sawyer, "Medicine and Christianity in the Modern World," in Martin E. Marty and Kenneth L. Yaux, *Health/Medicine and the Faith Traditions* (Philadelphia: Fortress, 1982), 133–60.

185 Samuel Hahnemann, *Organon of Medicine*, J. Kunzli and P. Pendleton, trans. (London: Victor Gollanz, !983).

186 Martin Albert and Bracha Mildworf, "The Concept of Dementia," *Journal of Neurolinguistics* 4, no. 34 (1989): 301–8. The way in which the etiology of dementia has changed over time: "One possible interpretation of these historical trends in the definition of dementia is that we are becoming more accurate in our understanding of the problem, i.e., that we are moving closer to the true definition of dementia."

187 This is one reason to choose not to focus on the wider term "dementia" throughout.

188 *The ICD-10 Classification of Mental and Behavioral Disorders.* See http://www.who.int/classifications/icd/en/.

189 Cheston and Bender, *Understanding Dementia*, 53.

190 The list is produced by the Alzheimer's Society. See http://alzheimers.org.uk/site/scripts/documents.php?categoryID=200362.

191 Tom Kitwood, "The Dialectics of Dementia: With Particular Reference to Alzheimer's Disease," *Aging and Society* 10 (1990): 177–96.

192 Cheston and Bender, *Understanding Dementia*, 67.

193 Glen Weaver, "Embodied Spirituality: Experiences of Identity and Spiritual Suffering among Persons with Alzheimer's Dementia," in Malcolm Jeeves, ed., *From Cells to Souls—and Beyond: Changing Portraits of Human Nature* (Grand Rapids: Wm. B. Eerdmans, 2004), 77–101.

194 Arthur Kleinman, *Patients and Healers in the Context of Culture: An Exploration of the Borderland between Anthropology, Medicine and Psychiatry* (Los Angeles: University of California Press, 1980).

195 Eileen Shamy, *A Guide to the Spiritual Dimensions of People with Alzheimer's Disease and Related Dementias: More than Body, Brain, and Breath* (London: Jessica Kingsley Publishers, 2003), 45.

196 Donald McKIm, ed., *God Never Forgets: Faith, Hope, and Alzheimer's Disease* (Louisville: Westminster John Knox Press, 1998).

197 David Keck, *Forgetting Whose We Are: Alzheimer's Disease and the Love of God* (Nashville: Abingdon Press, 1996).

198 Trevor Adams, "Kitwood's Approach to Dementia Care: A Critical but Appreciative Review," *Journal of Advanced Nursing* 23 (1996): 948–53.

199 Ibid.

200 Jonathan Franzen, "The Long Slow Slide into the Abyss," *The Guardian*, 15 December 2001; accessed on March 1, 2012, http://www. thelancet.com/journals/lancet/article/PII0149-6736(10)61286-X/fulltext.

Chapter 8

201 Arthur Kleinman, *Caregiving: The Soul of Care* (London: Penguin Random House, 2020).

202 James M. Houston and Michael Parker, *A Vision for the Aging Church: Renewing Ministry for and by Seniors* (Downers Grove: Intervarsity Press, 2011).

203 Genova, *Still Alice*, 98.

204 Robert Bogdan and Steven J. Taylor, "Relationships with Severely Disabled People: The Social Construction of Humanness," *Social Problems* 36, no. 2 (April 1989): 135–48.

205 Ibid., 139.

206 Ibid.

207 Ibid.

208 Ibid.

209 Franzen, "The Long Slow Slide into the Abyss."

210 Ibid.

211 Ibid.

212 Warnock, "A Duty to Die?" 25.

213 Ibid.

214 "Alzheimer Scotland Response to Baroness Warnock," accessed on March 1, 2012, http://www.alzscot.org/pages/media/Alzheimer_Scotland_response_to_Baroness_Warnock.htm.

215 Phillipa J. Malpas, "Do Those afflicted with Dementia have a Moral Duty to Die? A Response to Baroness Warnock," *New Zealand Medical Journal* (2009): 53–60.

216 Kitwood, *Dementia Reconsidered*, 19.

217 Stephen Post, *The Moral Challenge of Alzheimer's Disease: Ethical Issues from Diagnosis to Dying* (Baltimore: John Hopkins University Press, 1995), 3.

218 Ibid.

219 By "liberal cultures," I mean forms of liberal democracy, a system of democracy based on autonomy and individual rights and freedoms.

220 Kitwood, *Dementia Reconsidered*, 7.

221 Ibid., 47.

222 Ibid., 51.

223 E. M. Brody, "Excess Disabilities of Mentally Impaired Aged: Impact of individualized Treatment," *The Gerontologist* 25 (1971): 124–33.

224 Steve R. Sabat, *The Experience of Alzheimer's Disease: Life through a Tangled Veil* (Oxford: Blackwell, 2001), 93.

225 John Swinton, *Resurrecting the Person: Friendship and the Care of People with Severe Mental Health Problems* (Nashville: Abingdon Press, 2000).

226 Sabat, *The Experience of Alzheimer's Disease*, 94.

227 Julian C. Hughes, Stephen J. Louw, and Steven R. Sabat, eds., "Mind, Meaning, and Personhood in Dementia: The Effects of Positioning," in *Dementia, Meaning, and the Person* (Oxford: Oxford University Press, 2006), 287.

228 Rom Harré and L. van Langenhove, *Positioning Theory* (Oxford Blackwell, 1999).

229 Steve R. Sabat, "Positioning and Conflict Involving a Person with Dementia: A Case Study," in Fathali M. Moghaddam, Rom Harré, and Naomi Lee, *Global Conflict Resolution through Positioning Analysis* (New York Springer, 2008), 81.

230 Sabat, "Mind, Meaning, and Personhood in Dementia," 289.

231 Lisa Snyder, *Speaking Our Minds: Personal Reflections from Individuals with Alzheimer's* (New York: Freeman, 1999).

232 Sabat, "Positioning and Conflict Involving a Person with Dementia," 82; Snyder, *Speaking Our Minds*, 123–4.

233 Snyder, *Speaking Our Minds*, 123–4.

234 Sabat, "Positioning and Conflict Involving a Person with Dementia," 84.

Chapter 9

235 Thomas DeBaggio, *Losing My Mind: An Intimate Look at Life with Alzheimer's* (New York: Simon and Schuster, 2003), 88.

236 Ibid., 87.

237 Ibid., 7.

238 Robert Davis, *My Journey into Alzheimer's Disease* (Carol Stream, IL: Tyndale House, 1989), 53.

239 Betty Davis, *My Journey into Alzheimer's Disease*, 140.

240 For further development of the pastoral significance of lament in the face of suffering, see John Swinton, *Raging with Compassion: Pastoral Responses to the Problem of Evil* (Grand Rapids: Wm. B. Eerdmans, 2006), Chapter 5.

241 Aileen Barclay, "Psalm 88: Loving with Dementia," *Journal of Religion, Disability, and Health* 16, no. 1 (2012), 88–101.

242 Ibid.

243 Arthur Kleinman, "Caregiving: The Odyssey of Becoming More Human," *The Lancer* 373 (January 2009): 293.

244 Simone Weil, *Waiting on God* (London: Fontana Books, 1950), 76.

245 Ibid., 78.

246 DeBaggio, *Losing My Mind*, 7.

247 Alexander Nava, *The Mystical and Prophetic Thought of Simone Weil and Gustavo Gutierrez: Reflections on the Mystery and Hiddenness of God* (New York: University of New York Press), 31.

248 Weil, *Waiting on God*, 80.

249 Eric O. Springsted, *Simone Weil and the Suffering of Love* (Cambridge: Cowley Publications, 2010), 31.

250 Ibid., 45.

251 Weil seems to indicate that God really does abandon the person and truly is absent in the midst of affliction. Scripture, however, is filled affirmation that God does not abandon his people, even in the midst of affliction. Nevertheless, to *feel* abandoned is not particularly different from actually being abandoned.

252 For a deeper exposition of the concept of shalom, see John Swinton, *From Bedlam to Shalom* (New York: Peter Lang, 2000), Chapter 4.

253 Arthur Southland, *I was a Stranger: A Christian Theology of Hospitality* (Nashville: Abington Press, 2006).

254 The word in Greek is *philoxenos*, which means "stranger loving: being kind to strangers; being hospitable."

255 "An Anonymous Brief for Christianity Presented to Diognetus: The Mystery of the New People," Christian Classic Ethereal Library, 5.2–6, accessed June 1, 2012, http://www.ccel.org/ccel/richardson/fathers.x.i.ii.html.

256 Ibid., 5.6–11.

257 Cohen, in *Encounter with Mystery*, 156.

258 Ibid.

259 Ibid., 157.

260 Malcolm God Smith, "Through a Glass Darkly: A Dialogue between Dementia and Faith," *Journal of Religious Gerontology* 12, no. 3 (2002): 123–38.

261 Jean Vanier, *Becoming Human* (London: Darton, Longman & Todd, 1999), 33.

Chapter 10

262 Vanier, *Becoming Human*, 45.

263 James Woodward, *Encounter Illness* (Norwich, UK: Hymns Ancient & Modern, 2011), 54.

264 Albert Jewell, *Spirituality and Personhood in Dementia* (London: Jessica Kinsley, 2011), 45.

265 Alzheimer's Research UK, "Alzheimer's Research UK Launches as Public Dementia Fear Spiral," accessed Feb. 17, 1992, http://www.alzheimerresearchuk. org/news-detail/Alzheimer's- Research-UK-launch.

266 Luis Bunuel, in Joseph Ledoux, *Synaptic Self: How Our Brain Become Who We Are* (New York: Viking Press, 2002), 97.

267 David Keck, *Forgetting Whose We Are: Alzheimer's Disease and the Love of God* (Nashville: Abington Press, 1996), 32.

268 See Steven R. Sabat, "Capacity for Decision-making in Alzheimer's Disease: Selfhood, Positioning, and Semiotic People," *Australian and New Zealand Journal of Psychiatry* 39 (2005): 1030–5; quotation on 1030–1.

269 Keck, *Forgetting Whose We Are*, 43.

270 Christine Bryden and Elizabeth Mack inlay, "Dementia: A Spiritual Journey Towards the Divine: A Personal Review of Dementia," *Journal of Religious Gerontology* 13, no. 3, 4 (2003): 69–75; quotation on 71. The interior quotation is from Alzheimer's Disease International, 2002; accessed Feb. 2, 2002, http://www.alz.co.uk/.

271 Ibid., 72.

272 Ibid. The interior quotation comes from Bryden, *Dancing with Dementia: My Story of Living Positively with Dementia* (London: Jessica Kingsley, 2005), 153.

273 Peter Kevern, "Sharing the Mind of Christ: Preliminary Thoughts on Dementia and the Cross," *New Blackfriars* 91, no. 1034 (2009): 408–22.

274 Margaret G. Hutchison, "Unity and Diversity in Spiritual care." Paper originally presented at the Sidney University Nursing Society's First Annual Conference for Undergraduate Nursing Students in NSW (September 1997). accessed June 1, 2012, http://members.tripod.com/marg_hutchison/nuese-4.html.

275 Steven Sapp, "Living with Alzheimer's: Body, Soul, and Remembering Community," *Christian Century* 115, no. 2 (1998): 54–60; quotation on 60.

276 Ibid.

277 Malcolm Goldsmith, "Dementia: A Challenge to Christian Theology and Pastoral Care," in Albert Jewell, ed., *Spirituality and Aging* (London: Jessica Kingsley Publishers, 1999), 125–35, 129–31, adapted in Peter Kevern, "What Sort of a God is to Be Found in Dementia? *Theology* 113, no. 873 (May 2010): 174–82; quotation on 176.

278 See, for example, James W. Ellor, "Celebration the Human Spirit," in Donald K. McKim, ed., *God Mever Forgets: Faith, Hope, and Alzheimer's Disease* (Louisville: Westminster John Knox, 1998), 3, and in the same volume, Denis Dombkowski Hopkins, "Failing Brain, Faithful God," 37.

279 Kevern, "What Sort of a God Is to Be Found in Dementia?" 177.

280 Ibid.

281 David Keck's work, *Forgetting Whose We Are: Alzheimer's Disease and the Love of God,* represents by far the most developed and extensive theological exploration of dementia currently in print. This is a rich book, arising from his experience of his mother's dementia, reflected on from a broadly postliberal perspective underpinned by a Barthian theology of the Word. Thus, it treat God's sovereignty as 'non-negotiable,' focuses on the cross, and takes what it understands to be the traditional body of church doctrine as a given. Although Keck speaks of the suffering Christ, it is as an offering of human suffering to God and not a revelation of a compassionate God. His Christ offers us an "'Alzheimer's hermeneutic in which the displacement of self in listening for the Word of God. Keck's God is a loving and responsive one, waiting for our openness to the Spirit, but in the final analysis uncompromisingly impassible and sovereign, outside of and above the situation, not within it." See Kevern, "What Sort of a God Is to Be Found in Dementia?" 176.

282 Dietrich Bonhoeffer, *Letters and Papers from Prison,* Eberhard Bethge, ed., Reginal H. Fuller, trans. (London: Macmillan, 1953), 361.

283 St Augustine, *Confessions,* R. S. Pine-Coffin, trans. (London: Penguin Classics, 2002), X.8

284 Ibid., X.9.

285 Ibid., X.14, 16, 17.

286 Daniel Schachter, *Searching for Memory: The Brain, the Mind, and the Past* (New York: Basic Books, 1997), 16.

287 Ibid., 17.

288 Deborah Wearing, *Forever Today: A True Story of Lost Memory and Never-Ending Love* (London: Corgi, 2007).

289 Schachter, *Searching for Memory,* 17.

290 Quote in Ibid.

291 Schachter, *Searching for Memory.*

292 On the question of what it may be like to live without being able to forget, see A. R. Luria, *The Mind of a Mnemonist: A Little Book about a Vast Memory,* Lynn Solotaroff, trans. (Cambridge: Harvard University Press, 1986).

293 The point in quoting Keck is simply to suggest that his premise is wrong, not to directly dissociate his views with those of Singer.

294 Dallas Willard, "The Redemption of Reason," 1998. A transcription of an address given by Willard on February 28, 1998 at Biola University in La Mirada, California, at the academic symposium, "The Christian University in the Next

Millennium"; accessed Jan. 20, 1997, http://www.dwillard.org/aticals/artview. asp?artID=118.

295 Brevard S. Childs, *Memory and Tradition on Israel* (Naperville, IL: Alec R. Allenson, 1962), 33.

296 Ibid., 32.

297 Eugene H. Merrill, "Remembering: A Central Theme in Biblical Worship," *Journal of the Evangelical Theological Society* 43, no.1 (March 2000): 27–36.

298 Our identity is held in the memory of God is quite different from assuming that the soul is a natural entity that endure "under its own steam" into eternity. Only God is eternal, and only that which is eternal can bring that which is transient into eternal life. The Old Testament seems to express this point quite clearly.

299 Lisa Genova, *Still Alice* (London: Simon & Schuster, 2009).

300 Weaver, "Senile Dementia and Resurrection Theology," *Theology Today* 42 (1986): 447.

301 Ibid., 448

Chapter 11

302 Jean Vanier Quote: "The friend of time doesn't spend all ... https://quotefancy. com/quote/1453441/Jean-Vanier...

303 Tim Kearney, "Discovering the Beatitudes at L'Arche," *The Furrow* 35, no. 7 (July 1984): 460–4.

304 Jean Vanier, *Community and Growth* (London: Darton, Longman & Todd, 1979), 80.

305 Stanley Hauerwas, *There Is a Bridge*, DVD, accessed Sept. 1, 2007, https://www. imdb.com/title/tt1163888. This is a documentary focusing on the importance of continued communication with people suffering from Alzheimer's Disease.

306 Matthew 1:23: "The virgin will be with child and will give birth to a son, and they will call him 'Immanuel'—which means, God be with us."

307 St. Augustine, *The Confession of St. Augustine*, Albert Cook Outler, trans. (New York: Dover, 2002), 345.

308 Robert Jordan, "Time and Contingency in St. Augustine," John K. Ryan, trans. (New York: Doubleday, 1988), 394-417; quotation on 397.

309 Augustine, *The Confession of St. Augustine*, 345.

310 Sacks, *The Man Who Mistook His Wife for a Hat*, 37.

311 Ibid.

312 Sacks develops this point in some detail in his book *Musicophilia* (London: Picador, 2008), Chapter 29: "Music and Identity: Dementia and Music Therapy." See also Vernon Pickles and Raya Jones, "The Person Still Comes First: The Continuing Musical Self in Dementia, " *Journal of Conscious Studies* 13, no. 3 (2006): 73–9.

They argue that there is a residual musical self that remains even in the midst of severe dementia. This is an "enduring fragment" of who the person used to be.

313 Quoted from original version of Stanley Hauserwas's essay, "The Politic of Gentleness," presented at a conference hosted by the Centre for Spirituality, Health, and Disability at Aberdeen University.

314 John Goldingay, "Being Human," in Frances Young, ed., *Encounter with Mystery: Rejection on L'Arche and Living with Disability* (London: Darton, Longman &Todd, 1997), 138–9.

315 M. F. Egan, "The Sacrament of the Present Moment, " *The Irish Monthly* 65, no. 764 (February 1973): quotation on 111.

316 Thomas Merton, *Conjectures of a Guilty Bystander* (New York: Double day, 1966), 158.

Chapter 12

317 One can visit www. alz.org/10 signs.

318 Richard H. Gentzler, Jr., *Aging & Ministry in the 21st Century: An Inquiry Approach* (Nashville: Discipleship Resources, 2008), 36.

319 B. Reisberg, "Alzheimer's Disease," in J. Sadavoy, L. W. Lazarus, L. F. Jarvik, and G. T. Grossberg, eds., *Comprehensive Review of Geriatric Psychiatry,* vol. 2 (Washington, DC: American Psychiatric Press, 1996). This quote is from Harold G. Koenig and Andrew J. Weaver, *Pastoral Care of Older Adults: Creative Pastoral Care and Counseling Series* (Minneapolis: Fortress, 1998), 27–9.

Chapter 13

320 Richard E. Powers, *A Handbook for Spiritual Communities on Helping members with Memory Problem* (Tuscaloosa, AL: Bureau of Geriatric Psychiatry, DETA, 2007).

321 Koenig and Weaver, *Pastoral Care of Older Adults,* 21–3.

322 Robert S. Wilson, et al., "Loneliness and Risk of Alzheimer's Disease," *Archives of General Psychiatry* 64, no. 2 (2007): 234–40.

323 BBC News, "Loneliness Link with Alzheimer's," accessed Feb. 6, 2007, http://news.bbc.co.uk/1/hi/6332883.stm.

324 Ibid.

325 Janelle S. Taylor, "On Recognition, Caring, and Dementia," *Medical Anthropology Quarterly* 22, no. 4 (2004): 313–35.

326 Paul Ricoeur, *The Course of Recognition* (Cambridge: Harvard University Press, 2005).

327 Taylor, "On Recognition, Caring, and Dementia," 314.

328 Ibid.

329 Ibid., 319.

330 David Shenk, *The Forgetting: Alzheimer's: Portrait of an Epidemic* (New York: Anchor, 2003), 116–17.

331 Andrew Van Dam, "A Record Number of Folks Age 85 and Older Are Working," *The Washington Post* (July 5, 2018), accessed Feb. 26, 2020, https://www.washingtonpost.com/news/wonk/wp/2018/07/05/a-record-number-of-folks-age-85-and-older-are-working-heres-what-theyre-doing/.

332 Federal Reserve, "Report on the Economic Well-Being of U.S. Households in 2017", accessed May 25, 2018, https://www.federalreserve.gov/publications/files/2017-report-economic-well-being-us-households-201805.pdf.

333 "Working Later in Life Can Pay Off in More than Just Income" Harvard Health Publishing), accessed June 6, 2018, www.health.harvard.edu/staying-healthy/working-later-in-life-can-pay-off-in-more-than-just-income.

334 Christopher Quinn, "I Am Going to Work until God Tells Me Not to: Need or Desire for Keeping Record Number of Older Workers on the Job," *Houston Chronicle* (Aug. 8, 2019), Money/Retirement., B5.

335 Ibid

336 The Center for Retirement Research at Boston College was established in 1998 as part of the Retirement Research Consortium.. https://crr.bc.edu/data/public-plans-database. The Public Plans Data website is developed and maintained through a collaboration of the **Center** for **Retirement Research** at **Boston** College, the **Center** for State and Local Government Excellence, and the National Association of State **Retirement** Administrators. Access the Public Plans Data website

Chapter 14

337 R. Kane, J. Outlander, and I. Abrass, *Essentials of Clerical Geriatrics*, 5th ed. (New York: McGrew Hill, 2004).

338 Koenig and Weaver, *Pastoral Care of Older Adults*, 17.

339 Ibid., 18.

340 Zachary Zimmer, Carol Jagger, Chi-Tsun Chiu, Mary Beth Ostedal, Florencia Roja, Yasuhiko Saito, "Spirituality, Religiosity, Aging, and Health in Global Perspective: A Review," SSM: Population Health 2 (Dec. 2016): 373–81, accessed Dec. 1, 2018, https://www.sciencedirect.com/science/article/pii/S2352827316300179. Religious attendance has been shown to buffer the need for and length of hospitalization (Koenig, et al., 1992, 1998). There is also strong evidence of a connection between religiosity and mental health (Musick, Traphagan, Koeing, & Larson, 2000).

341 Christian Koenig and Uschi Konig, "Examination of Blood Samples of the Eurasian Otter (*Lutra Lutra*)," *IUCN Otter Specialist Group* 15, no. 2, 68–127,

accessed Oct. 12, 1998, https://www.iucnosgbull.org/Volume15/Konig_Konig_1998.html.

342 Ibid.

343 National Institute of Health, "Dealing with Dementia: When Thinking and Behavior Decline," Special Issue: Seniors, accessed Nov. 12, 2018, https://newsinhealth.nih.gov/special-issues/seniors/dealing-dementia. From the article, "Symptoms of dementia can include problems with memory, thinking, and language, along with impairments to social skills and some behavioral symptoms." Several factors can raise your risk for developing dementia, including aging, smoking, uncontrolled diabetes, high blood pressure, and drinking too much alcohol.

Chapter 15

344 T. R. Elliott, M. Parker, and L. Roff, "Family Caregivers and Health Care Providers: Developing Partnerships for Continuum of Care and Support," in *The Multiple Dimensions of Disability* (New York: Springer Press, forthcoming).

345 The idea that most families abandon their loved ones to nursing home is a myth. Most of families go through enormous hardships are extra ordinary committed to continue caring for their loved ones at home.

346 Lisa Gwyther and Maryann Matteson, "Care for the Caregivers," *Journal of Gerontological Nursing* 9, no. 2 92–5, accessed Feb. 9. 1983, https://www.healio.com/nursing/journals/jgn/1983-2-9-2/%7Badd6cda7-4be9-4bf4-bddd-133b5ed4542e%7D/care-for-the-caregivers. Caregivers often are surprised by how well the client adjusts and by how much more loving they can be when they are able to sleep and are not responsible for providing all of the physical care.

347 Lauren Austin and Holly Gershbein, *Love, Loss and Dementia: Stories about Our Parents with Dementia and a Validation of Your Journey* (Scotts Valley, CA: Create Space Publishing, 2018), 112. Holly and Lauren share with the reader their personal experiences of caring for aging parents with dementia. Reading this book is almost like sitting down with a caring friend who offers practical advice to help you through a challenging time. I found this book to be helpful as I try to care for elderly parents in a loving and respectful way.

348 Rabins, et al. (1990).

349 Koenig and Weaver, *Pastoral Care of Older Adults*.

350 Melanie Haiken, "How to Be a Good Caretaker, and Take Care of Yourself, Too," *Parade* (Dec. 23, 2016), accessed Dec. 22, 2020, https://parade.com/533756/melaniehaikencaringcomsenioreditor/caregiver-bootcamp-drawing-the-line/. "It gets you stuck, and it becomes a barrier to making the hard decisions that need to be made," says Los Angeles-based geriatric consultant, Jennifer Voorlas.

351 Melanie Haiken, "A Plan for Caring," *Parade* (September 2018): 12.

352 Dominic Cellitti, Protect Finances, "Future for Those with Cognitive Impaired Decline," *Houston Chronicle* (March 2019): SS7.

353 Frena Gray Davidson, *The Alzheimer's Sourcebook for Caregivers: A Practical Guide for Getting Through the Day* (New York: McGraw-Hill, 1994). The author is director of SHACTI (Self-Help Alzheimer's Caregiver's Training and Information), a fact-based, hands-on guide for those caring for in-home Alzheimer's patients. The purpose is to discuss how to deal with stress and difficult behaviors, how to find outside help, and how to nurture your own well-being.

354 Ideas for such preparation are discussed in more detail in, "Caregiving: The Twenty-first Century's Greatest Test of Character," in James M. Houston and Michael Parker, *A Vision for the Aging Church: Renewing Ministry for and by Seniors* (Downers Grove: IVP Academic, 1922), 196.

355 John Bowlby, *The Making and Breaking of Affectional Bends* (London: Tavistock, 1979).

356 Tessa Perrin, "Occupational Need in Severe Dementia: A Descriptive Study," *Journal of Advanced Nursing* 25 (1997): 934–41.

Chapter 16

357 Ross T., "Lion's Mane Mushroom aka Yamabushitake—Brain Food, Potential Fat Burner," *Researched Supplements* (Jan. 20, 2021), accessed Aug. 8, 2021, https://www.researchedsupplements.com/lions-mane-mushroom-yamabushitake. Yamabushitake mushrooms are eaten in Japan and China. The ethanolic extract of Lion's Mane has been shown in clinical trials. A new clinical study says "RediMind" can improve memory by 51% in 30 days.

358 UT Southwestern Medical Center, "New Insights into Alzheimer's", accessed July 10, 2018. https://utswmed.org/medblog/new-insight-into-alzheimers/. Scientists at UT Southwestern's O'Donnell Brain Institute have made a discovery that could change how and when doctors detect Alzheimer's—and it could also lead to more effective treatment for people living with dementia. Dr. Marc Diamond, Director of the Institute's Center for Alzheimer's and Neurodegenerative Diseases and a leading dementia expert, led a team to discover the exact moment that a healthy brain protein becomes toxic. The quote is his word after his discovery.

359 Researchers at UT Southwestern Medical Center have pinpointed the "Big Bang" of Alzheimer's disease. Published in the *Journal of eLife* (2018).

360 "New Insights into Alzheimer's." Read the full story here: https://www.utsouthwestern.edu/newsroom/articles/year-2018/genesis-of-disease.html.

Chapter 17

Conclusion

Appendix A

361 John Swinton, *Dementia: Living in the Memories of God* (London: SCM Press, 2012), 40.

Appendix B

362 Koenig and Weaver, *Pastoral Care of Older Adults.*

363 Tom Kitwood, *Dementia Reconsidered: The Person Comes First* (Buckingham: Open University Press, 1997), 19.

364 Tom Kitwood, 'The Dialectics of Dementia: With Particular Reference to Alzheimer's Disease," *Aging and Society* 10 (1990): 177–9.

365 Clive Baldwin and Andrea Capstick, *Tom Kitwood on Dementia* (Maidenhead: Open University Press, 2007), 74.

366 Baldwin and Captick, *Tom Kitwood on Dementia,* 74.

367 Ann C. Homer, et al., "Diagnosing Dementia: Do We Get it Right?" *British Medical Journal* 297 (October 1998): 894–6.

368 Baldwin and Capstik, *Tom Kitwood on Dementia,* 75.

369 Kitwood, *Dementia Reconsidered,* 62.

370 Andrew Sixsmith, John Stilwell, and John Copeland, "'Rementia': Challenging the Limits of Dementia Care," *International Journal of Geriatric Psychiatry* 8, no. 12 (December 1993): 993–1000.

371 Dennis Greenwood, "A Review of Dementia Reconsidered: The Person Comes First,'" *European Journal of Psychotherapy and Counseling* (1988): 154–7.

372 L. S. Caddell and L. Clare, "The Impact of Dementia on Self and Identity: A Systematic Review," *Clinical Psychology Review* (February 30, 2010): 113–26.

373 Hans S. Reinders, *Receiving the Gift of Friendship: Profound Disability, Theological Anthropology and Ethics* (Grand Rapids: Wm. B. Eerdmans, 2008), 21.

374 Swinton, *Dementia: Living in the Memories of God,* 92.

375 Ludwig Wittgenstein, *Philosophical Investigation* (Oxford: Blackwell, 1995).

376 Owen C. Thomas, "Interiority and Christian Spirituality," *The Journal of Religion* 80, no. 1 (2000): 41–60; quotation on 56.

377 The social nature of the mind is implicit even within Descartes' dictum, "I think; therefore I am." Who is the "I" that is thinking, and where is he? It appears that he is necessarily and inseparably connected to an "I." Presumably the "I" resides in the world of persons and is open to the types of contexts and influences that have been highlighted. We have no knowledge of any other world or any other way of being in the world. If the "I" is in the world, then the mind cannot simply be within the "I."

Appendix E

378 Elsevier, "The Cost of Alzheimer's Disease in China (2018)," *Alzheimer's Disease* 14, no. 4 (April 2018): 483–91.

379 Ray Kwong is a freelancer, blogger, and tweeter.

380 Peter Fuhrman, "Alzheimer's Is China's Biggest Future Health Problem," *Seeking Alpha* (June 6, 2017), accessed June 12, 2017, https://seekingalpha. com/article/4079071-alzheimers-is-chinas-biggest-future-health-problem-and-biggest-healthcare-industry. Alzheimer's is the fastest-growing, major fatal disease in China. Today there are at least 9.5 million diagnosed sufferers in China with perhaps as many cases undiagnosed.

381 The University at Buffalo is a premier research-intensive public university, a flagship institution among New York state universities and its largest and most comprehensive campus. UB's more than 28,000 students pursue their academic interests through more than 300 undergraduate, graduate, and professional degree programs. Founded in 1846, the University at Buffalo is a member of the Association of American Universities.

Printed in the United States
by Baker & Taylor Publisher Services